Your Guide to E-Health

Peter Yellowlees is Director of the Centre for Online Health, and Head of the Department of Psychiatry at the University of Queensland. He is an internationally recognised expert in health information technology and is in regular demand as an international conference speaker, giving more than 30 presentations world-wide each year for the last few years. He has published more than 90 scientific articles and book chapters, including many on e-health, co-authored one book and received well over $1 million in research grants. His full academic curriculum vitae is available at the website for the Centre for Online Health at http://www.coh.uq.edu.au. This site, which has been driven by Professor Yellowlees, receives heavy international traffic and is being promoted by the World Bank as one of the best health/IT sites in the world.

Professor Yellowlees is on the editorial board of the *Journal of Telemedicine and Telecare*, is the Chair of the editorial board of *Telehealth International*, and is on the clinical advisory board of DoctorGlobal.com. He is a regular reviewer for other journals and features in several educational videos and films. He has been the Director of Queensland Telemedicine Network since its inception in 1995. This is the most extensively used videoconferencing health network in the world.

Professor Yellowlees is involved in a series of exciting and leading-edge research programs, taking health-care services to patients in their homes, and preventative health education programs to students in schools, as well as to their families. He still practises part-time as a psychiatrist and is a strong believer in patients having access to information at any time and anywhere.

Your Guide to E-Health

Third Millennium Medicine on the Internet

Professor
PETER YELLOWLEES
Director, Centre for Online Health
University of Queensland, Australia

University of Queensland Press

First published in electronic form 2000 by University of Queensland Press
Box 6042, St Lucia, Queensland 4067 Australia

www.uqp.uq.edu.au

This edition 2001

Typeset by University of Queensland Press
Printed in Australia by McPherson's Printing Group

Distributed in the USA and Canada by
International Specialized Book Services, Inc.,
5824 N.E. Hassalo Street, Portland, Oregon 97213–3640

ISBN 0 7022 3220 3

CONTENTS

ACKNOWLEDGMENTS

Your Guide to E-health was written with the help of a great many people. First I would like to thank the many anonymous patients who taught and enthused me about the possibility of providing therapy online, and who led to me exploring the many possibilities of the Internet outside the field of psychiatry. I would never have become interested in this area if patients had not been so accepting of "seeing" me through a variety of electronic technologies since about 1992. I have had a great deal of support for my academic interests from my colleagues at the University of Queensland, in particular Professor Bryan Campbell and Professor Peter Brooks, as well as several colleagues in the Department of Psychiatry, especially Dr Gerard Byrne, who covered my normal work role while I was writing and researching.

Dr Ace Allen, past editor of *Telemedicine Today*, has been enthusiastic and supportive, and has helped significantly with his incisive comments on the manuscript. Al Zuckerman, from Writers House in New York, was also extremely encouraging, as well as appropriately critical in his reading of various drafts of the book, as was my agent, Margaret Kennedy.

Rosemary Spencer spent long hours improving my writing style and editing chapters. She made many valuable suggestions about the book and taught me much about the process of non-academic writing. Matthew Rickard assisted with excellent research and advice, always delivered with professional efficiency. Sheila Cleary and Trish Buckley assisted with secretarial support and cheerfully formatted my inexpertly typed drafts.

Finally my family: Jo, my wife, and Georgina and Charlotte,

my daughters, have put up with my rather overwhelming obsession for this topic, usually with tolerance and good humour, despite my odd predilection for turning on the computer at antisocial times of the day and night. My ultimate aim has always been to make a difference in the world and to develop ways in which patients can more easily access good-quality health care. They understand that and their love and care is greatly appreciated.

PREFACE

Welcome to "e-health"! This book has been written for people who want to use the internet to improve their health. It is written in a practical way to allow you to understand and select the type of health information or practitioner that is right for you. I've tried to put a human face on the amazing technologies that are becoming available and to show how we can benefit from them.

It is not a "hi-tech" book. It won't explain the intricacies of the Internet, or even how to log on. There are already many other books and manuals that do that and you should consult them as necessary.

Instead, *Your Guide to E-health* will explain how the Internet can be applied to your problem or situation. There is no similar book on the market for health consumers, although there are a number aimed at health professionals which deal with specific technologies, mainly computers.

In each chapter you will find case examples based on true situations which have been modified to protect identities. There are also checklists and self-assessments that you can use. Each chapter stands alone and deals with an entirely separate issue. The book's aim is to be a practical information source about e-health, with web addresses, references and practical hints on the best use of the Internet.

This book is written for you and you should treat it as you wish. Underline the sections that you find most useful. Write comments in the margins. Make your own notes as you read. Crease and fold the pages at important sections for easy reference. This book should not remain in pristine condition. It will probably end up being a reflection of you. Dip in and dip out of it! Read and re-read certain chapters or sections of special interest. Move from chapter to chapter. Think about the case examples and how they apply to you. Use the book as a work manual not just for conventional reading. Try the exercises on rough paper, or gather some friends and family around and try them as a group to see how they relate to you. Give it to friends that you think might find it helpful, or to colleagues, or to your doctor or therapist if you have one. Don't just leave it on the shelf after the first read. Leave it lying around where you'll see it and pick it up again!

Finally, please do not hesitate to send feedback and your suggestions for improvements for future editions to me at P.Yellowlees@mailbox.uq.edu.au

CHAPTER 1

E-HEALTH — A REVOLUTION IN HEALTH CARE

I recently put the word "health" into the Alta Vista web search engine. The search returned 27 million webpages where the word "health" was mentioned. I followed up with other words. "Money" found 9.6 million pages, "sex" 10.2 million and "Microsoft" 9.7 million. What an amazing statement about the popularity of health on the net — almost as many mentions as sex, money and Microsoft put together!

The business of e-health on the Internet is expanding rapidly. Forty-three per cent of United States Internet users utilise the Internet for health information and health care. Around the world in the year 2000 it was estimated that about 100 million people sought health information on the internet. Despite many recent "dot com" crashes business still sees the health-care sector as a particularly attractive industry that will benefit from web-based technologies because of its enormous size, inefficiency and information intensity. Moreover, the health-care industry is particularly fragmented, with a large number of participants, including general practitioners and primary care clinicians, specialists, institutions (public and private hospitals and diagnostic companies), health funds, pharmaceutical companies, retail pharmacies and, of course, patients.

John Chambers, from Cisco Systems, was recently quoted as saying that "the Internet waits for no-one". How true is his statement. We know that the radio took 30 years, and the TV 15 years, to build an audience of 60 million people around the world. The Web won 90 million people in under three years and hasn't looked back. Countries such as China, with its aggressively supportive policies regarding the Internet, and regions such as South America and the Indian subcontinent, with their large populations and economic bases, are likely to become very significant powers in the Internet world over the next decade. Some commentators have even suggested that Chinese might be the most common language on the Internet by 2010.

Many forces are making the practice of e-health advance rapidly.

- Consumers are spending more of their own income on health, with an estimated increase in cost of 2.5 per cent to 3.5 per cent per year as the population ages.
- Consumers are being encouraged to take more responsibility for their health, and to know more about treatments offered to them, their effectiveness and the track record of the individual provider or medical team offering the treatment.
- It is known that conventional health services can cause many unintended injuries or complications, and government task forces in the United States, Europe and Australia have all strongly recommended more information technology involvement in the healthcare system to reduce errors and mistakes.
- Health practitioners are becoming increasingly computer literate. The recent Practice Incentives Program from the Australian Federal Government has led to approximately 70 per cent of GPs now being online, while in America about 85 per cent of doctors now access the Internet, mainly for email. There are several major commercial organisations offering doctors their own homepages, and the culture of health is changing rapidly in Australia and America. In particular, it is now well understood by both patients and doctors that patients can drive their care through accessing good-quality information. Doctors are learning to respond in what will be a more market-focused system.
- There are a series of highly publicised and funded Internet health portals that have recently been developed. These include

Healtheon/ WebMD in the United States, as well as the Health Communication Network, and three other similar organisations in Australia. Major publishing companies, such as the Murdoch and the Fairfax organisations, are developing substantial health-care Internet programs, as is Microsoft.

- The Australian health-care industry is worth $47 billion per annum, with the American equivalent industry being 25 times bigger, and in this environment one of the major problems is a lack of reliable health content, or guides to health, on the Internet.

Your Guide to E-health is written to help fill that need, to inform consumers of the advantages of the Internet in health. But it is also to assist people using the Internet, particularly when interacting directly with doctors or other health-care professionals, to ask the right questions to ensure they are not being fooled. It will help people with the sorts of health problems illustrated throughout the book, like in the following examples:

I picked up the phone with a feeling of dread. "Please Doc, you've got to talk to my husband. I can't stand his drinking anymore. There's no way we can get in to see you. You're 300 miles away and anyway we can't leave the farm during lambing. I'm desperate. Last week he was drunk and I thought he was going to shoot us all. He keeps talking of suicide and how we're going to make ends meet."

A call from another patient. "I'm scared to leave the house. When I go out I feel like I'm going to have another heart attack. My chest pain just won't go away. I feel I have to always be near the phone to be able to call for help. I don't want to die. My kids think I'm daft and my husband's fed up. He's been great, doing the shopping and running the children around; but there's only so much he can take. I need some way of monitoring my heart that won't mean I have to call you all the time."

The Internet and email

Today e-health mainly involves the Internet and email, which are rapidly taking over from the phone and videoconferencing (often called telemedicine), the technologies that have been used to deliver online health in the past. In the near future the capabilities of the phone and video will be fully available on the Internet and most distant health communications will use this single platform. This recent wave of interactive technology has meant that patients and their clinicians are able to communicate in more ways, and with more effectiveness, than could have been imagined even ten years ago. And the pace of change is escalating. It is estimated that the speed and power of computer technology is doubling every 18 months.

There are three main types of clinical interactions on the Internet: therapist/patient, therapist/therapist, and particularly patient/patient. Patients are using the Internet to help each other. Widespread access to the Internet and email has enabled great improvements in clinical and teaching services worldwide. At the University of Queensland's Department of Psychiatry the webpages are designed with a series of hot links. These links enable patients to access websites easily all over the world. They offer good-quality information on issues ranging from depression and suicide to child abuse. (The website is www.psychiatry.uq.edu.au.)

But the Internet is not a place for the unwary. Sir Robert Baden-Powell, when he dreamed up the Boy Scout motto "Be prepared" many years ago, wasn't thinking of the Internet, but his warning is appropriate for Internet users. When looking for a doctor through the Internet, be wary, suspicious, hesitant. Thoroughly check out therapists or websites to ensure that they meet professional standards and are not money making, "fly by night" operations. It is interestingtomakeregular checks on suspicious-looking sites, say every fortnight or so. It is amazing how frequently they suddenly shut down or move — not the sign of a reputable operation. As long as you are careful, the Internet is a great place to find information, although it is not yet a great place to connect with individual therapists. So, as with any new adventure, go cautiously!

The changing face of health care

A new millennium — a revolution in health care. Within ten years visiting a doctor or therapist over the Internet will be as natural as attending a medical centre. Within the safety and convenience of our own homes we'll be able to speak to health professionals, access information on our health and receive support from groups of people with similar problems. Wireless videophones will be commonplace and we will be able to live in a virtual environment if we wish, able to contact our doctor, order groceries from the supermarket or set the security system in our home from wherever we are.

Our population is an ageing one with "baby-boomers" demanding better-quality and more home-based health care. Governments are trying to reduce the escalating cost of health care by cutting back in various ways, including closing down hospitals.

But it won't be long before they realise that it is not only cheaper to treat people at home online, but patients can also become more involved in their own care. With a touch of a switch, patient, GP, specialist and health nurse can be brought together. Care will be more accessible and of better quality. Heath professionals will be more accountable and patients better informed.

The net is widening

Already 45 per cent of American homes contain a computer and most hospitals now have videoconferencing facilities. Well over 250 million people around the world use the Internet regularly, many of them exclusively for email. Fifty per cent of adults in the United States have used the Internet, compared with 23 per cent in 1997. It is forecast that within a few years 500 million people will be Internet users. The Internet as a health-care centre, accessible to millions of people around the world, will be an awesome reality.

The call from patients for more input into health matters is growing. For example, the last decade has seen an enormous rise in the number and power of self-help health interest groups. These groups have recognised the power of mass communication and are using the Internet to provide information to their members and to gather support for their causes through user groups and bulletin boards.

At the same time computers are becoming more affordable. You can now buy a good-quality home computer for less than $1500 and the cost is falling nearly as fast as online technologies are improving.

E for expectations

The Web offers an amazing combination of immediacy, global reach, personalisation and specialisation. It has led to our expectations changing for basic service and product delivery. We now expect 24-hour global access, speed, do-it-yourself resources, mobility, personalisation and customisation, a large range of services and products, as well as the ability to pay online. In short, more choice and access, more empowerment. The convergence of technologies such as the phone, the wireless, broadband Internet access and digital TV is rapidly increasing the power and availability of information. (Why else would Time Warner and America Online have recently merged?) The excitement caused by this convergence is reflected in the exponential growth of use of the Web, where uptake indicators are defying gravity. For some time, Internet traffice has been doubling every hundred days, and the recent broadband shifts are increasing the speed of the Web by 50 to 100 times. Even Europe, which has been relatively slow in the race to join the Internet era, is predicted to have by 2004 one in three of its connections by broadband. As the .com, .org and .nets are joined by domain names such as .tv, with 24-hour streamed television on demand, it is mind-bending to think of the overall effect of the Web on global society.

Feeling the byte

In the United States health-care professionals make almost 1000 million home visits every year. Most of the patients are elderly or chronically ill. More dramatically the home healthcare market in the United States, which was estimated to cost $34 billion in 1996, will cost $66 billion by 2003.

But while home care is expensive, it is still cheaper than in-patient care. The current cost of in-patient accommodation alone in the United States is $820 million a day, before any treatment costs are added. That's $3 for every American every day! If just one person in every 200 could be treated outside an institution there would be an annual saving of nearly $2 billion. Similarly, another $1 billion could be saved by reducing the number of people in nursing homes by just 5 per cent, that is, one person in twenty. Obviously, it will be much cheaper for patients to be properly cared for in their own homes using e-health.

The move toward home-based e-healthcare will not, however, be driven solely by the need to cut costs. The rapidly aging generation of "baby boomers" will insist on more and better-quality home care and community services. As a member of the so-called "indulgent" and "demanding" generation, I have no intention of being hospitalised except under the most dire circumstances!

It's *your* health chart

How often have you wanted to read what your health professionals have written about you? Through a shared electronic medical record you'll not only be able to read what your doctor or therapist has written but you'll also be able to check that it is accurate and even contribute to it yourself.

This health homepage will contain all your health records. You will be able to make notes in it and collaborate with all types of health-care professionals. Because it is on the Internet it will be accessible to you wherever you are in the world. It will be linked to health information, videomail, email and a range of related technologies that will allow you to see your own X-rays, pathology results, even your surgeon's operating notes. Within about ten years the following scenario will be commonplace:

> *I've had a night of terrifying palpitations so, before going to work, I decide to seek reassurance from my doctor. I go to my home communications system and, via the individualised touch screen, press the videophone icon to speak to my doctor's receptionist, Mary.*
>
> *Almost immediately Mary comes on screen via a secure high-speed video Internet connection. She compares my online diary with my doctor's and asks if I would prefer an appointment in person, either at the clinic or at my home, or by video, either to*

my home or via my laptop at work.

I decide to leave a note describing my symptoms in my shared electronic medical record for my doctor to look at when she comes in from her early morning home visits. She will either email or videomail me back if she thinks I should see her sooner than my scheduled consultation.

Keying in my password, I access my own record via the secure directories and write a short note about my symptoms. When I use the word "palpitation" it is highlighted as hypertext. I hit the hotlink and download a patient information sheet on "palpitation", developed by a university in England and recommended by my doctor. While I have my electronic medical record open, I scan back and check what my doctor wrote the last time we met. I am pleased to see that her treatment plan is based on the clinical guidelines developed for my heart condition recommended by the physician I saw some months before.

Before going to work I take a few minutes to read the information on "palpitation" and remind myself of some simple techniques I can use to keep my heart rate steady during the day.

While this sounds futuristic, everything in the scenario is actually possible today. The individual technologies need only to be integrated and speeded up. This will happen in the next few years.

Home care — the way of the future

Online therapeutic techniques are about to change radically the face of home care. The following scenario is already happening in pilot programs around the world and uses equipment that costs only a few hundred dollars at each site.

"The tea smells wonderful, darling." Sylvia's voice comes from the bedroom. "Can you get me my medication — my pain is awful this morning — it's so hard to get my joints moving." Peter shuffles across the kitchen to the cupboard and takes out the medication

dosette containing his wife's daily medication, each dose carefully worked out by Carol, their home nurse, on one of her regular visits. He takes the morning pills for his wife's arthritis, pain and depression through to the bedroom. She's in so much pain and unable to move about much any more. He's thankful that he is still reasonably fit and can help her at home.

He'd been surprised at how easily she had taken to using the small video camera which now sat above the TV set. By using a telephone link they could see and talk to Carol and their doctor through the video camera and their own television.

Since Carol had brought the system they had seen a lot more of her. She used to come three times a week but was always in a hurry. It seemed she spent more time driving than visiting. Now she only visited the house twice a week but they usually had at least two other video sessions with her, which Sylvia really seemed to look forward to. He couldn't understand why she dressed up and put on her make up for the TV sessions but it seemed to do her good!

It was also wonderful that their daughter, who lived too far away to visit regularly, had bought a similar set-up. Seeing her on the screen was so much better than speaking on the phone and, of course, it was lovely seeing the grandchildren!

Sylvia had always been a very independent person and refused to go to hospital. To monitor her pain and disability she agreed to fill in a weekly questionnaire of her symptoms which Carol scanned into her medical records. This way Sylvia's doctor could monitor how she was feeling.

Once a week, during one of her visits, Carol arranged a weekly TV conference link with the doctor. This had greatly improved the communication between everyone.

This scenario shows how online health technology can both improve the quality of health care and save money. E-health allows people to be treated in their homes and facilitates better communication between all those involved in the caring process. Studies have shown that home-health nurses average five to six home visits per day when working exclusively from their cars in the traditional manner. If they used online health technologies they could probably make three home visits each day and six to eight video visits.

Potential users of e-health

Almost anyone with a chronic illness, and many people with non-life-threatening acute illnesses, can be helped by e-health. Clearly people who are acutely ill require urgent face-to-face assessment, and interventions such as hospitalisation may be necessary as a life-saving measure.

Electronic consultations are happening across international borders, to remote rural regions in many countries, to prisons and nursing homes, and to the physically or psychiatrically disabled within their own homes. Other beneficiaries of e-health include people who are frequently on the move or on holiday. Some people simply prefer e-health to conventional face-to-face approaches, or use it as an adjunct to their normal care, in particular to gain more information about their condition or to contact others involved in self-help or support groups. Consultations using broadband, usually satellite, technologies have been held with people on ships, in space and on aeroplanes, as well as in geographically isolated areas, especially in America, Canada, Australia, China and other parts of Asia.

For deaf people the Internet is a special bonus. Unable to communicate by telephone, they are able to use the Internet to communicate with their friends or their doctor over great distances. The same applies to the many people around the world who have aphasia, a condition usually caused by strokes, where people cannot speak because of damage in their brain but fully understand everything that is going on around them.

Now they can communicate online, despite being physically unable to speak.

People involved in self-help or support groups who want to get to know other sufferers or to learn more about their illness are important users of the e-healthcare. The Internet offers an extraordinary choice of self-help, support and information options for patients and families around the world. It is possible to find all manner of treatments, some bizarre, such as "urine therapy" where you supposedly benefit by drinking your own urine, mainstream alternatives such as homeopathy, acupuncture and meditation, and conventional approaches, especially huge amounts of information on medications.

And finally there are those who are involved in the prevention of disease, in research, in administration, and in community-focused public health activities. In Malaysia planning is well under way for the Multimedia Supercorridor — a national health program using online techniques to focus on education and illness prevention. This is the way of the future.

Some people already live in "wired communities". Whole towns, such as Telluride in the United States, have been given online access as an experiment. Early evidence suggests that the online world can be extremely supportive, particularly for those who are lonely. It also seems that meeting people over the Internet may encourage more face-to-face interactions and a wider network of friends. With my unusual name I have already found several relatives on the Internet that I didn't know existed, and have been delighted to meet them later face to face.

But how do we relate to each other online?

Relationships online

Internet relationships have been explored by Esther Gwinnell, MD, a psychiatrist from Oregon, in her fascinating book *Online*

Seductions — Falling in Love with Strangers on the Internet (1998). She demonstrates clearly that it is possible to develop effective and empathic relationships online, but she also outlines the potential pitfalls of such romances. She believes that it is important to understand more about this phenomenon:

> *Falling in love over a machine? Many people find the idea humorous or even ludicrous. Yet it is happening, and psychotherapy patients are reporting this phenomenon to mental health professionals worldwide. It has become important to explore the ways in which people fall in love on the Internet, and to understand the similarities and the differences between them and relationships formed in person.*

Although there is an abundance of excellent and accurate information available online, there is also some that is horrendously biased and inaccurate. Unfortunately, it can be hard to differentiate between the two unless one has some core knowledge of the subject, especially as some of the most potentially damaging information is produced in a highly professional way. So how does one differentiate between the good and the bad? The easiest way is to check whether the therapists or website writers have published their work in international and reputable journals. This is not difficult to do. To determine these people's credibility, and the credibility of their health websites, ask yourself these questions:

- Are the doctors, or other health professionals, actually the people they say they are?
- What are their qualifications and do they practise in an ethical manner in accord with clearly laid down standards?
- Are you sure they are not going to take your money and run — probably to another homepage to fool more people into parting with their money?

Education and illness prevention are the strongest online

modalities at present, with accurate information about health problems recognised as being therapeutically beneficial to patients, significantly accelerating recovery. But you have to be able to assess the online doctors, and their websites, in ways that are critical yet reasonable. This book will give you straightforward guidelines on how to do this.

Will e-healthcare change therapeutic relationships?

The major problem with online relationships is developing a realistic view of your therapist or doctor that is not clouded by the electronic wizardry. The clinician has the same problem but also has to break through similar barriers created by what I call our "e-persona". There is developing evidence that we tend to act and communicate rather differently when we are online, particularly via email where no visual contact is made. The same is true in videoconferencing, where therapeutic relationships also seem to be different even though the patient and doctor can see each other. Charles Zaylor MD, a psychiatrist at Kansas University Medical Centre and one of the most experienced telepsychiatrists in the United States, told me:

> *I have become more direct with patients using telemedicine. I don't beat about the bush. It is somehow a more practical relationship that focuses very much on what people are doing in their lives, and how I can help them with good advice.*

In a similar way, my online experience has changed the way I work with patients that I see in my normal practice as well as those I talk to online. My therapeutic goals and objectives are now more overt and specific. I'm more open and honest with patients about what I believe are their problems and the solutions and, in particular, I give them far more health information.

What makes an effective online doctor?

E-doctors still need all their traditional talents, especially empathy, warmth, flexibility, understanding and honesty. But they need more than that. They need to understand the issues brought about by their own, and their patients', online persona. This is an extra, complicating feature of the relationship.

E-therapists need better communication skills, not only in an individual setting but also in groups. They must be able to project their personality in a similar manner to actors. Some people seem personable and friendly face to face, but projected onto a screen they portray as much presence as a dead fish. Although media training can help, such therapists are probably better off minimising their online work.

Of course some people never discover what type of online persona they have. These people are terrified of technology, particularly computers, and develop panic attacks and a sudden desire for a long walk in the country at the very thought of an online interaction.

Telephobias and tele-addictions

We all respond differently to new technologies. Feelings of helplessness or anger against computers or other technologies can lead to technophobias or telephobias, which have many causes, mostly social and cultural. They affect mainly females, but occur in varying degrees in up to half the population. Mark Brosnan, in his book *Technophobia* (1998), has gone as far as to suggest that such reactions are a "legitimate response to technology". It has been suggested that telephobia may be age-related. However, the large number of retired people who enjoy using computers does not support this. This is important, as it is the elderly, through home care, who will be one of the sectors of society to benefit most from e-health.

Solutions to telephobias are examined in detail in Chapter 8, as is the rapidly emerging problem of tele-addictions. Most people in western societies will have read of cases of tele-addiction or know of people afflicted by it. As with any new experience, there is always a group of people who go overboard in their enthusiasm. The online world provides an escape for many people, but it can interrupt normal social activity, family relationships and psychological development. The latter is an especially important issue for adolescents, who can develop computer "nerd"-like lifestyles.

Internet activities are especially addictive. Surfing the net is rather like gambling — one always expects to find the ultimate homepage in the next few minutes, just like one hopes to hit the jackpot. When a surfer does find a great website, possibly after hours of surfing frustration, their gambling instincts are reinforced and they carry on looking for the next "big win". Email users often have a tendency to check their mail several times a day "just in case" there is something urgent. Evidence is now emerging that email may interfere with work and home efficiency — and enjoyment of life — if it is not carefully managed.

Fortunately there are solutions to the tele-addictions. If you are worried that you, or someone you know, might have a tele-addiction or telephobia, use the brief self-assessment questionnaires that are included in Chapter 8. They will indicate your risk of having, or developing, these disorders. In time, as online technology and therapy become increasingly common, people will learn to handle these types of difficulties. And that brings us back to the future.

The future

What will happen to e-health over the next ten, twenty or fifty years, and how will the relationships between patients and their therapists change as a consequence? No-one can be certain how they will change, but change they will.

Warner Slack MD (1997) has predicted that all medical services will move out of hospitals to places of patient convenience and that hospitals as we know them today will disappear. He calls their replacements, which would be within walking distance for many patients, “clinhavens”. These facilities would be outpatient-based and have sufficient information technologies and clinicians available to enable them to provide comprehensive care.

Over the next decade clinicians and the health system will be overtaken by the Next Generation Internet (NGI), also known as Internet 2, which will be up to a thousand times faster and more powerful than the present Internet. The NGI is already at an advanced stage of development and will be available soon.

The NGI will drive the changes to health care over the next ten years. More and more e-healthcare systems will be developed and embraced by patients and clinicians alike. Technologies will merge, and e-health will become part of normal health practice, so that many people will be treated with a combination of face-to-face and e-health approaches. While these changes are inevitable, the main obstacle to their acceptance will be cultural and attitudinal inertia within the health system, as clinicians struggle to change their work practices and therapeutic relationships. It is crucial that patients know what is possible, so they can make informed choices, and so that any resistance to the widespread use of e-healthcare is broken down.

I believe that e-health, and the Internet, will radically change the whole health system and lead to much better health for all of us. Care in all its guises will be more accessible and of a higher quality, while health professionals will be more accountable to better-informed patients. Doctors will have their own homepages where they will detail their experience, their continuing professional development, their licence details and the results of their treatment. Surgeons will detail their infection rates, oncologists their cure rates, psychiatrists their patient-rated outcome measures, and most doctors their patient-satisfaction scores.

The parallel developments of the Internet and the consumer movement will create massive changes in health care. These will lead to a more accessible, reactive, fair and friendly health system which is increasingly individualised and focused on the needs of patients.

There will be improved communication between doctors and their patients, with more emphasis on collaboration and long-term therapeutic relationships facilitated by these new technologies. Face-to-face care and e-care will merge and make care more accessible for all, and eventually global health-care systems, crossing boundaries, continents and time-zones, will emerge. The roles and training of doctors and other health professionals will change as they work not only differently but more effectively.

Health education and disease prevention will finally become central to the provision of health care and health research will gather momentum with the increased availability and accessibility of information.

More people will be looked after in their homes at the expense of hospital and institutional care, and patients and health professionals alike will have an enriching and fascinating experience travelling the path of change together for the ultimate good of all.

What an exciting future for patients and clinicians alike!

CHAPTER 2

WHO WILL BENEFIT?

It is fascinating to reflect on the changing cycle of health care over the past two centuries. Two hundred years ago if you were literate and rich and wanted to see your doctor you would probably have written to him describing your symptoms. Your doctor, who worked on his own, would have written back prescribing treatment which may or may not have included leeches or bowel washouts. Confidentiality was not an issue. Your health problems were often very public knowledge! Doctors didn't carry out physical examinations, because not only were they often socially unacceptable but doctors struggled to interpret the results.

However, from the mid 1850s there was an increasing understanding of the importance of specific physical and psychological symptoms and the health-care system has gradually changed. From a highly distributed, open, community-based process, people began to be institutionalised in hospitals, and the confidentiality of individual health records became increasingly important. In the last 50 years there has been a gradual move back towards community care with the realisation that community-based health promotion and prevention activities are more effective in the long run than expensive hospital care. This change is being accelerated by the online technologies which allow health information to be distributed widely and easily. And so we have just about gone full circle as we move back towards a distributed, community-based system. The difference is that this time we have more education, more information and more privacy.

But what about the changes that have occurred broadly

across our society in recent times? As a baby boomer I find it astonishing that most first-year university students today wouldn't know who killed JR. In fact, who was JR? For them Michael Jackson has always been white, the SS *Titanic* was never lost and AIDS has always existed. They were born the year the Walkman was invented, they do not remember the Cold War, they have never seen black and white television, and they have experienced only one Pope.

This is the world we live in. It's changing more rapidly than at any previous time in history. The way we deliver health care is changing just as rapidly.

Covering the territory

"Circuit riding" is a normal part of many people's lives. Lawyers, salespeople, marketers, engineers and teachers regularly travel great distances to service rural centres. It's hard work and disruptive to family life. Most give it away after a few years, leaving younger colleagues to take up the challenge.

For years I was a psychiatrist "circuit rider". I regularly flew out from my home town of Broken Hill with the Royal Flying Doctor Service to hold clinics in towns hundreds of kilometres away. One of the places in the vast Australian outback I used to visit regularly was White Cliffs, 600 kilometres from the nearest state capital of Melbourne and 300 kilometres from Broken Hill. White Cliffs is a small opal-mining town built on chalk where the summer temperatures are routinely over 40°C and most people live underground in excavated modern-day caves.

Over the years my understanding of the town and its people grew, but so did my frustration. My patients never seemed to be unwell on the day I visited; they always seemed to get sick between times. This meant that when I arrived they were either better, often following telephone consults, had left town to receive treatment elsewhere, or had become so ill and anxious or paranoid, through having received no treatment, that they'd gone into hiding and couldn't be found at all!

If I'd been able to access the online technologies that are available now I could have "seen" patients between clinics and treated them in the early stages of their illnesses. Through the Internet I could have provided training and supervision to the town's health staff. My clinic visits would have been more productive, as I could have spent more time with patients instead of running around town trying to find people who were untreated and unwell.

In future the most common users of e-health will undoubtedly be those patients who integrate virtual care with their normal face-to-face care — they will see their doctors in the surgery and in cyberspace. This is what I do with my own patients at present, and is what is being offered by Internet consulting services such as http://www.doctorglobal.com. There are certain groups of patients who will find e-health particularly helpful whether they integrate it into their usual face-to-face care or not.

People who are unable to access relevant health expertise in their community, especially the geographically isolated

Most health professionals live in major cities — often where they were brought up and trained. Comparatively few people from rural regions study health programs at universities, and most of those who do, choose to stay on in the cities rather than return to the country. This means that many communities have inadequate health expertise, while the centre of cities may have "too many" experts.

Isolation in all its forms is a major cause of human distress. Human beings are inherently social creatures and rural dwellers suffer more from depression and alcohol abuse than their city counterparts. Generally, rural people's access to e-health is more limited because the telecommunications infrastructure needed to support telemedicine or good Internet access is not always available. Fortunately, this situation is changing, and within a few years fibre-optic cables, wireless systems and satellites will make online technologies widely available.

People who prefer to receive care, monitoring and support at home instead of in hospitals or other institutions

In America the national annual expenditure on home care in 1997 was $42 billion. Between 1989 and 1996 the number of home-care agencies grew from 11,000 to over 20,000 and the cost of home-care visits increased from $70 million per annum to $306 million. At the same time hospital costs are also escalating, and world-wide attempts to reduce these costs are being made by discharging patients as early as possible. This is known as managed care, an intellectually dishonest term if ever there was one. In the United States this policy of early discharge for financial reasons has reached extraordinary levels, where patients can virtually only stay in some hospitals if they are actively and continuously suicidal or if they cannot walk.

Clearly, cost is one of the drivers behind the move to increase home care. Equally importantly, aging baby-boomers are now starting to develop a personal interest in home care as the generation ages and they take a growing interest in taking responsibility for their own health care. In the light of these changes it is inevitable that patients will demand tele-home-care services once they understand how effective they can be.

Perhaps the greatest benefit of e-care is that people can be treated in their own homes. The leading telemedicine journal, *Telemedicine Today*, devoted its entire December 1997 issue to "tele-home health", highlighting a number of fascinating projects. Richard Wootton, Professor of Online Health at the University of Queensland, Australia, and an international pioneer of telemedicine, has reviewed the case notes of 1700 patients being nursed at home in the United States and the United Kingdom. He estimates that up to 45 per cent of home nursing visits in the United States and about 15 per cent in Britain could be made via telemedicine, and in the future by the Internet. This suggests that billions of dollars could be saved.

Equally importantly, those involved in current home-health programs report almost universal patient satisfaction with the services. In *Cybermedicine* (1997) Warner Slack MD states:

> *Gradually all medical services will move out of the hospital to places of convenience to the patient … Using interactive computing in their homes, patients themselves will manage medical problems … Doctors will make house calls. Clinicians and patients will know each others' names and will work together as friends.*

So what are some of the applications of e-health in the home? There are so many that I will highlight just two: the world-renowned Kaiser Permanente home-nursing service run by the charismatic and energetic home-care nurse Barbara Johnston, and an Italian home-monitoring service.

The Kaiser Permanente program started in 1996 and now incorporates over twenty home-care monitors being used by a nursing team at any one time. This particular home-care system is used mainly for patients with chronic physical illnesses — heart and lung disease, terminal cancer, severe diabetes — but people with chronic depression, anxiety and major social and psychological disorders are also treated. The program has markedly reduced the "down" time that nurses spend in physically travelling between patients, has increased their productivity from 5–6 visits a day to 15–20 video visits a day, and has also reduced the number of patients who have been hospitalised.

An Italian telephone-mediated home-monitoring service has been functioning since 1987. It helps meet the medical, especially cardiac, social and psychological needs of 25,000 home-bound patients, using a telephone call centre and home-monitoring system. One of the fascinating outcomes of this service has been a much lower than expected suicide rate for that group of patients, as they have gained so much support and confidence from knowing that their medical problems, mainly heart disease, are being carefully monitored.

People on ships, aeroplanes, submarines or spacecraft or in places without access to conventional health care

The world is already dotted with satellites that form a global communications network. Originally developed for the defence and media industries, the network is now increasingly being used for health purposes. One such commercial company is Inmarsat which has 10 satellites and more than 100,000 mobile earth stations. Currently it is the only company providing global communications for distress and safety, as well as having commercial applications at sea, on land and in the air. More companies and organisations will undoubtedly enter this market soon. It is now possible to communicate with patients and monitor their vital signs and psychological status on aircraft, oil rigs, ships and in the most remote parts of the world and send the information to relevant hospitals or, in particular, military health-care institutions.

North Sea oil rigs and platforms

A paramedic on an oil rig wearing a headset with a miniature video camera, a small TV screen and a two-way audio link examines a patient. The data is fed via satellite and land lines to the Accident and Emergency Department at the Aberdeen Royal Infirmary in Scotland where the relevant specialist advises on the patient's condition.

Sea Med

Sea Med is a program run from the Cedars Sinai Medical Centre to provide health assistance to the many people who are at sea. Sea Med estimates that there are over 6,000 super or mega private yachts, none with any medical capability. There are also over 100 cruise line companies carrying on average 400,000 passengers with an average age of 52 and variable medical support. Within the Merchant Marine Navy around the world there are a further 40,000 ships with over 300,000 crew members at sea every day. Minimal or non-existent medical care is provided for these people. Of course the large number of naval fleets at sea do often have very significant medical support on board. Overall, well over 1 million people are at sea every day who could potentially be treated by e-health. Transmitting via a giro-stabilised satellite antenna mounted on ships, Sea Med carries out medical consultations with people aboard ships through high-quality video imagery. Each ship is equipped by Sea Med with medical equipment and a drug inventory, very much like the Royal Flying Doctor Service has equipped outback homes in Australia since 1927.

Climbers on Everest

Following the tragic deaths of 12 climbers on Mt Everest in March 1996, an expedition in 1998 successfully incorporated a trial of e-health technologies. The climbers were equipped with monitoring and telecommunications devices which successfully transmitted back much useful health information. Several climbers also swallowed capsules that transmitted information on their core body temperature back through base camp to Yale–New Haven Hospital. It is hoped that the knowledge gained about the effect of extreme climates on humans will prevent further deaths.

Spacebridge to Russia

The National Aeronautics and Space Administration (NASA) and the Russian Space Agency have been developing a medical education and consultation program since 1996 through the Spacebridge to Russia program. It is expected that this will eventually allow patients and clinicians at a number of centres in the United States and Russia to interact in real-time audio and video over the Internet. This will be in use even before the introduction of the much faster Internet 2, which should give people in the most remote areas access to the best specialists and medical centres.

Groups that need special interpreting skills that aren't available locally

Deafness is very common. In the United States 0.5 per cent of the population, or over 1 million people, are unable to use a telephone even with a hearing aid. The introduction of care on the Internet opens up a whole new world of communication possibilities for these people. Support groups have flourished on the web, and several doctors in America and Australia now use “signing” via telemedicine to communicate with the deaf. These sorts of services will be transferred to the Internet once broadband access is more widely available.

People who prefer e-care to face-to-face help, or who use it as an adjunct to their normal therapy

There is no doubt that some people prefer to answer computer-based rather than face-to-face questions. And many will answer a computer program more honestly than when asked the same questions by a doctor. This applies particularly to questions that might be seen as embarrassing or personal.

A classic example is child sexual abuse. Up until approximately 15 years ago, child abuse was believed to be very rare. In fact, when I was training as a doctor in the 1970s it was not mentioned in the curriculum at all. Yet we now know that sexual abuse of children is tragically very common. Given that in the past most doctors were males and most victims were females, it isn’t surprising that the female victims didn’t report abuse to their male doctors. If there had been other ways to collect data in those days apart from face-to-face interviews, the extent of the problem might have come to light much earlier.

Impotence is another example. Relatively few males admit to this problem in an interview, especially if the interviewer is young, attractive and female. Yet impotence clinics that advertise in the media and set up fairly anonymous services are overwhelmed by clients, especially since the advent of Viagra, which sells in huge quantities on the anonymous Internet via web pharmacies. People find it difficult to admit their concerns and fears to others face to face.

Some people simply find relating to other humans a chore, preferring the relatively unemotional environment of the computer. In earlier times these people might have become hermits, living out their lives in isolated caves, or entered monasteries or nunneries to avoid too much human contact. Becoming a shepherd or farming an isolated patch of country were other alternatives. Today such people tend to be labelled "avoidant", "schizoid" or "socially phobic". They often find it difficult living in our varied and busy society, but, despite their difficulty communicating face to face, they still have strong emotional needs and are likely to benefit greatly from the increased accessibility to health professionals online.

People who want to get to know other sufferers, or who wish to learn more about their illness

Loneliness can be particularly distressing. It is possible to be lonely in a crowd or in the centre of a bustling city. Loneliness is especially miserable when one is unwell, confused, uncertain or distressed. It is a medical fact that mortality rates are higher among socially isolated or lonely people and that this risk factor is independent of other well-known risk factors such as smoking, drinking, social class and level of physical fitness. It is not known why this is, but most humans do have an intense need for other humans, for relationships, for friends, and these things are good for our health. So when we suffer from chronic illnesses such as asthma, heart disease, arthritis, cancer or depression we tend to try to find other sufferers to communicate with and learn from. This has been difficult in the past. The Internet, in particular, is dramatically changing all this, enabling sufferers to meet one another and gain support and help from those who understand their situation best, their fellow sufferers. There are a remarkable number of online support groups and many will be accessible throught the websites listed in the appendix to this book. If you have a mental-health problem, consult Dr John Grohol's comprehensive listings in his excellent book, *The Insider's Guide to Mental Health Resources Online.*

Physically or psychiatrically disabled people who find it difficult to leave their homes

This is the classic case of "if the mountain won't come to Mohammed, then Mohammed has to go to the mountain". In the past, people who were paraplegic, had severe disabling arthritis or suffered extreme agoraphobia often missed out on useful therapies because they couldn't get to a therapist.

The addition of e-care to home-care initiatives for these people will make a substantial difference.

Institutionalised populations, such as prisoners, or elderly people in nursing homes

E-health systems, at present using telemedicine but soon to go on the Internet, are now regularly used in American prisons and are often linked to academic medical centres. Examples of prison online health systems are found in Texas, North Carolina and Ohio. Here e-health is used for almost all types of health care, allowing paramedics in the prisons to work with medical specialists to diagnose and treat prisoners. Online health care allows prisoners much better access to high-quality health professionals than would otherwise be possible and at a much reduced cost to the institutions. Without these services it would be hard to deliver the constitutional right of prisoners to quality health care.

Nursing homes are another area where e-care is being developed. In America and Australia a series of low-end videoconferencing systems using ordinary phone lines (POTS — Plain Old Telephone System) are being introduced into nursing homes to give the occupants immediate access to their treating health staff at any time. Interestingly, many of the residents' children are also likely to buy the equipment, which costs only about $400, so they can keep in visual contact with their parents. Imagine how much pleasure this will bring elderly people and their families. These systems will rapidly become redundant, however, when the Internet can routinely be used for video communications combined with information access, allowing e-care to be much more effectively delivered.

Travellers, holiday makers, or those who want to keep in contact with their doctor after they or the doctor have moved away

A colleague of mine from England recently married his Australian fiancee in Brisbane. Unfortunately his parents weren't able to come out to the wedding from England as one of them had had a stroke. No problem. My colleague hooked up his laptop computer and included them in the wedding by videoconferencing to England. The wedding went well, his parents heard him take his vows, and they were able to videotape the entire ceremony back in England to keep as a lasting memory. Although they couldn't taste the wedding cake or kiss the bride, they were able to share in the special occasion.

I have on several occasions agreed to follow-up patients by telephone when they have moved to other states and are "between" therapists. Nowadays when I go overseas patients email me if they need to contact me while I am away. In the past the only options for continuing care were by phone or post, but today email is commonly used. After all, why shouldn't you be able to access your usual doctor wherever you are in the world? And why shouldn't doctors be able to communicate easily with other clinicians in the event of an emergency? We expect TV news to bring us live interviews with people all over the world. We should expect the same level of service in the health domain. The only reason we don't is that people don't realise it's readily available. It is!

People involved in prevention, research, administration or community public health activities

The best way of improving our health is to prevent problems before they arise. Research shows that 6–14 year olds are highly receptive to messages about healthy living. At this age patterns of unhealthy or health-threatening behaviour haven't become bad or lifelong habits. The Internet offers tremendous opportunities in this regard as most schools in developed countries are now connected, as are more than 45 per cent of homes. Children love education delivered electronically, as long as the programs are interactive and stimulating, and their teachers, supervisors or parents confident and knowledgeable. We have the opportunity to introduce lifelong protection, through early education of our children, against melanoma (skin cancer caused by excessive exposure to the sun), infectious diseases, particularly HIV and AIDS, obesity and various addictions. Online health prevention programs for children are currently being developed at the Centre for Online Health (www.coh.uq.edu.au) and will become available over the next few years.

Researchers will also reap the benefits of e-health. In the past valuable data was often consigned to wastepaper baskets because everyone communicated verbally and made notes on paper. As shared electronic records are introduced, valuable epidemiological data about health and illness patterns will be more easily available. We might even be able to discover whether mobile phone users do actually run an increased risk of developing brain cancer if we are able to study enough people through these means.

In the long run we all benefit

In the long run we all stand to gain from e-health even if we're not personally involved. This is because the development of e-healthcare will lead to a general upgrading of health services. At present, doctors tend to treat individual illnesses, but online care will lead to an increased emphasis on continuity of care, health promotion and illness prevention. There will be an attitude change in both patients and clinicians. These important issues will be discussed in Chapter 7.

Malaysia, with its policy of Vision 2020, has set itself the goal of "becoming a fully-developed, mature and knowledge-rich society by the Year 2020". To do this it is developing the Multimedia Supercorridor. This is an area of about 750 square kilometres south of Kuala Lumpur, which is embedded with an extraordinarily high bandwidth digital communications infrastructure to link to centres of information, manufacturing and service provision across the country. The Malaysian government plans to integrate technological infrastructure and social systems with electronic health care as one of their "flagship applications". This initiative aims to keep people in a state of "wellness" through integrating seamless health information and cyberspace help services. The clinical programs will be supported by a series of educational programs for doctors and other Malaysian health-care professionals. Hence the aim is not just distant medical consultations, but to develop genuine primary prevention programs across all areas of health. This will include, for the entire population, individual "lifetime health plans". It will be a major social change. Singapore has gone

one better, with plans to have every home in the country linked to the Internet.

At the other end of the scale, Nepal, a very poor country of 22 million people, immense mountains, isolated communities and very few doctors, is also starting to use the Internet to provide professional health education to its very isolated practitioners, to support them, and to keep them up-to-date with the latest medical advances.

Who shouldn't use e-health?

This is difficult to answer as there are no absolute contraindications to the use of e-health and every clinical situation should be assessed individually.

You may have concerns about the online doctor's professional competence, ethics or qualifications. If your "therapist" believes that a one-year course in navel gazing from the College of Emotional Harmony in Never Never Land is sufficient to practise psychotherapy over the Internet, I suggest you tell them to go straight back to Never Never Land. Always remember that Internet and email therapies may be offered by almost anyone. The message is "buyer beware". Check out the doctor. Follow the advice in Chapter 6.

If you are uncomfortable with the online approach, and reasonable alternatives are available, then use them. If there aren't any alternatives, you will need to deal with your discomfort. It may be that telephobia is the problem and ways of overcoming this are discussed in Chapter 8. Using the equipment shouldn't be a problem. With the appropriate support and encouragement anyone can learn how to handle it. Obviously if you can't get access to the necessary technology e-health is not an option.

Your health problems may be too serious to be treated online (for example acute medical, surgical or psychiatric emergencies). Patients with these problems are often assessed online, but face-to-face assessment and treatment and often hospitalisation may well be urgently required.

In a crisis you should be able to obtain help locally if your online doctor is not contactable. Ideally, of course, your online doctor and your face-to-face doctor would be the same person, with you making the choice as to whether you "see" them face-to-face or via the Internet. Competent doctors will always make certain that emergency back-up is available locally for the times they are away or unavailable. (Of course this might not be possible if you live in an extremely remote area.)

Would e-health suit you?

The following eight-point questionnaire will help you decide if you, or members of your family or your friends, would benefit from e-healthcare. Try it out.

- Do you have access to the Internet?
- Would you feel comfortable communicating electronically?
- Are you geographically isolated from the health services you need?
- In the event of your not being able to contact your online doctor in a crisis, do you have access to a therapist or doctor in your local community?
- Do you have a physical or psychiatric disorder that makes it difficult for you to leave your home or community to receive treatment?
- Would you prefer to be treated at home or in your local community rather than in an institution?
- Would you like to communicate with people with the same disorder as you?
- Would you like more information about your disorder?

The more positive answers you have given, the more likely

you are to benefit from e-health. Remember, there are no absolute contraindications apart from not having the right equipment to access the Internet.

CHAPTER 3

TODAY'S SERVICES

Innovations in health tend to go through a typical cycle. When a breakthrough is announced everyone is ecstatic and the new discovery is hailed as the cure-all to end all cure-alls. As with Viagra, everyone wants a slice of the action! But inevitably there follows a period of disillusionment; there are problems, the common cold hasn't been cured, early enthusiasts now wouldn't use the new wonder drug on their dog! But in time the innovation reaches the third and final stage and finds its niche market.

The Internet is a classic example. Developed originally by the military for defence purposes, the Internet was then used as a communication tool for university academics, and during the 1990s went through a period of uncritical acceptance. It is now supported at last by some evidence of effectiveness, although still not nearly enough. We are beginning to use it more critically, particularly with the advent of recent global viruses, such as the "love bug" of May 2000 which wiped out hundreds of thousands of hard drives world-wide, creating a damage bill of billions of dollars. Most people who start using email still use it massively and uncritically before working out what it is useful for and what merely wastes time. The telephone is the same. The onset of adolescence, especially in females, seems to be accompanied by a passionate urge to spend most of the day on the phone. In time this phase passes and the phone is subjected to more rational use.

Over the next few years videoconferencing will increasingly be provided through the Internet. This won't change the sort of health care offered online, but it will make interactive e-health-care far more available, and to more patients. But enough of the future. Let's look quickly at the past, and the development of the Internet.

The technology

If you want to know anything about the Internet, how it works, what it is, the latest developments, a glossary of terms, the major players, listings of relevant books and links to an unbelievable number of other sites, simply go to www.whatis.com. If you haven't got ready access to the Internet, go to an Internet café or a library to look this one up. The visual explanations, in particular, are fantastic and it'll save you hours of hard slog.

In brief, the "net" is owned by you as a public collaboration. It grew from a small research defence network in the United States developed to function even if a large portion of it was destroyed by a nuclear war. When you link from your computer via a modem to an ISP (Internet service provider), you connect to their server (essentially a large computer attached to the global telecommunications network). You use your browser (a small program on your computer — usually Netscape or Microsoft Internet Explorer) to select the address (the URL — uniform resource locator) of the site you wish to visit. The site is situated on another server anywhere in the world also attached to the public network. This process is called "surfing".

The most widely used part of the Internet is the World Wide Web (the "Web") which allows you to link by hypertext, highlighted or coloured text, to other sites around the world. The most commonly used single application on the net is email, which for many people has virtually replaced letter writing.

To access the net, all you need is a reasonably new computer, a modem and an account with an ISP who will usually provide the computer software you require. It will cost you under $1500 including the cost of the computer to start up and a few hundred dollars per year to connect. This has to be one of the best-value buys in the modern world. Connection through your cable TV operator, or via satellite, will often give you much more rapid access, but may cost more.

Clinical uses of the Internet — information and learning

The Internet is the largest and most disorganised library in the world. It contains massive amounts of good information on every subject under the sun, especially health. However, it also contains huge quantities of misinformation, which at best could be described as biased or warped. A couple of Christmases ago I decided to look for some historical information about "Santa Claus" for my daughters. Fortunately they were not looking over my shoulder, because all I discovered were the remarkable sexual activities apparently enjoyed by modern day "Santas".

Before we can benefit from the Internet we have to solve the problems of information quality and information overload. Efforts are currently being made to create good-quality sites that deliver "guaranteed", accurate health information. Examples include the National Library of Medicine in the United States (www.ncbi.nlm.nih.gov), OMNI (http://omni.ac.uk) and NHSNet (www.nhsdirect.nhs.uk) in the United Kingdom and Healthinsite (www.healthinsite.gov.au) in Australia. A more comprehensive Internet classification and coding system, as well as the development of better search engines to "mine" information, are required as part of the long-term solution to this major problem. Only then will doctors and patients be able to effectively obtain good-quality decision-support information within the time alloted for a typical online or face-to-face consultation.

Despite this problem, and contributing to it, there are increasing numbers of health portals available on the Internet which focus on a particular topic (such as epilepsy), a particular country (such as Australia), a professional organisation (such as the American Medical Association) or an entire business network such as (Compuserve or America Online). The aim of these portals, unless they are being set up for mischevious reasons, is to ensure that the hypertext links from the portal connect only to sites that provide good-quality information. The key to finding good information on the Internet at this stage is to find good portals. A selection of the best health portals and search engines can be found in the appendix. Throughout this book you will find Internet addresses of sites of reasonable quality. Unfortunately, though, as sites are constantly changing, there's no guarantee that they will stay that way.

How common is health information on the net?

It is estimated that there are over 100,000 websites primarily devoted to health, and about 40 per cent of people who use the Internet use it for health-related reasons. There is a simple way of estimating how much information on health there is on the Web. Just go to a very broad search engine, such as Alta Vista, and put in a simple and common term that relates to your area of interest. Then count the number of webpages returned to you by the search engine where your word is picked up.

I did this for a series of common words and names and found millions of pages that reported using these words:

Sex	10 million	Beatles	4 million
Money	9 million	Pamela Anderson	0.1 million
Microsoft	10 million	Bill Gates	0.3 million
God	4 million	Jesus	2.5 million
The Bible	3 million	Coca-Cola	0.3 million
Tax	4 million		

I deliberately chose these words because they are either in common use in the English language, or commonly reported to be important issues on the Web. It is fascinating that "sex", "money" and "Microsoft" all turned up around the same number of pages. "God", the "Bible", "Jesus" and "tax" all came in at around the same levels of interest and popularity, along with the "Beatles". Rather to my surprise, "Coca-Cola", perhaps a more specific search word than some of the others, and "Bill Gates" were much less popular, but still were mentioned over 300,000 times, while "Pamela Anderson", who has often been reported as being the single most effective salesperson on the Web, via her sex marketing profile, featured on only about 100,000 pages.

So what about health-related words? All I can say is that they were amazingly common. The term "health" which admittedly can be used in a variety of ways, and doesn't necessarily relate purely to medicine, was shown on 27 million websites, as common as "money", "sex" and "Microsoft" combined. Mind you, I thought I'd have a look at the first website that came up under the health search term and found myself in a highly pornographic, voyeuristic site! But that is the Web, and it shows how careful you have to be, and how much overlap there is on general searches by topic. Here are the number of webpages found on Alta Vista that mention some common health words:

Birth	6 million	Doctor	2 million
Death	5 million	Medication	0.3 million
Disease	3 million	Nurse	0.6 million
Hospital	3.5 million	Physician	1 million
Medicine	5 million	Therapist	0.2 million
Patient	2 million	Alcohol	1 million

Compare these terms with the non-health items mentioned

earlier. "Birth", "death" and "medicine" are all more commonly mentioned than "God", the "Bible" and "tax". "Doctor" and "patient" appear about as commonly as "Jesus", and "alcohol" gets three times more mentions than "Coca-Cola"!

Sure this is not high science. It is only a simple example of the amount of potentially relevant health information on the Web. But it's convincing.

Links with like-minded individuals

The Internet allows people with similar interests, passions or problems to connect, interact and communicate with each other, generally via email, after finding out about each other through conventional advertising in the press or via websites, bulletin boards, chat groups or Internet search engines.

One of my patients is a good example of this. Distressed by unusual symptoms of depersonalisation, where she feels detached from her body, she has gained a great deal of support and information from the Internet. Surfing the net she discovered a specific research program on depersonalisation in Europe, and after completing assessment protocols for the project by email she was invited to take part in the research.

Contact with groups of fellow sufferers through the Internet has made her feel less alone and she has also learned of several unusual therapeutic options to reduce the distress caused by her symptoms. We don't know whether they will work yet, but the fact that they have been recommended by other sufferers has been most helpful to her.

Individual or group services through an Internet doctor

This is cowboy country at present. Relatively small numbers of patients are currently being formally treated on the Internet by qualified professionals, despite the hype and self-promotion of other so-called professionals. However, I'm certain that it won't be long before recognised treatments and consultations become widely available on the Internet. Advice on selecting a reputable Internet doctor is given in Chapter 6.

One of the best Internet medical services, and one of the few being set up with a strong ethical and clinical base, is http://www.doctorglobal.com. This site is an example of what is to come, of how common email consultations will be, of how simple virtual consultations can be. And how a group of health professionals, mainly doctors, can combine to offer quality e-health services in many countries and for a range of purposes. Doctor Global, set up by a New Zealand general practitioner, Dr Tom Mulholland, has eleven online clinics: General, Sexual, Heart, Travel, Nutrition, Allergy, Occupational Health, Mental Health, Asthma and Sports Medicine. There are already considerable numbers of consultations being performed by the qualified medical staff who subcontract their services to Doctor Global, and whose photographs and professional credentials are shown on the site. Sites such as this which offer accountable, quality, ethically sound health services are still uncommon.

Other health activities on the Internet include bulletin boards, discussion groups and mailing lists for health professionals and patients to communicate and exchange information. These are unlikely to change much in the next few years, but they will become more sophisticated and interactive, with more real-time chat events, and will incorporate video as well as the written word.

Continuing education will be a major growth area for professionals, with more interactivity and voice/picture combinations becoming available over the Internet. Such programs are beginning to be offered using the new technology of videostreaming, sending videos directly through the Internet so that they can be watched from home at any time. Some professional associations have even been developed specifically for the online world. The International Society for Mental Health Online at www.ismho.org is one such organisation. It has been formed to promote mental-health activities and services online and to formulate standards and credential checks for clinical practice online.

Buying health-care products

This is perhaps the most high profile and most clinically problematic area. The sale of medications via the Internet is hugely profitable for those companies that are involved, but it is a major ethical problem, and if it continues in a completely unregulated way has the potential to cause much harm. Viagra is a drug that has sold well on the Web. It is used to treat impotence, and many men who take it are afraid to discuss their problems with their doctor — it is much easier to get on the Internet and order the medication direct. The problem is that a drug like Viagra should only be taken after consultation with a doctor, because it has significant side effects, particularly cardiac, and also interacts with other medications, with significant potential for harm. Although much prescribing on the Internet is done via reputable doctors and pharmacy chains, much is not. It is essential that patients do not use the net as a short cut, often via dubious websites, to obtain potentially dangerous drugs.

"B to C", or Business to Consumer, and "B to B", Business to Business, are the two main models of Internet business interaction. Both involve the sale of products, whether they be wheelchairs, medical hardware, information or medications. Whatever the product the Internet is an amazing e-commerce medium, and with the health sector valued at 14 per cent of the US Gross Domestic Product, there is a lot of value for those who wish to sell health-related products. There are many "health information" sites whose main object is to sell products, often dubious or useless, to consumers or health professionals. They often suddenly link you with a range of "natural products" or with sites that encourage spending on a wide range of related products. Even more worrying for the unwary are the sites that send "cookies" (small embedded computer programs) to your computer, which can identify your surfing habits, and consequently your interests, to the originating site, so that they may more easily target their sales pitch to you in the future. Watch out for the emails full of great ideas for you to spend your money on! Buying health products is like buying anything else — take advice from others, do not spend large amounts of money impulsively, and make sure that the product you are buying is of good quality, works effectively and is value for money.

History of the computer and the Internet

A comprehensive history of computing would have to include the Chinese abacus, Charles Babbage's "analytical engine" of 1834 and the many mechanical calculators built in the 19th and early 20th centuries. However, the first real electronic computer was Turing's "Colossus", used by the British military from 1943 onwards to help break codes used by the German army in World War II. High-level programming languages such as FORTRAN were introduced from the mid fifties, and the development of integrated circuits and operating systems in the early sixties led to huge gains in computational power and efficacy. In the seventies microcomputers and workstations were introduced as the miniaturisation and integration of computer components proceeded. Microsoft was founded in 1975, Apple in 1977 and by 1978 more than half a million computers were being used in the United States. The IBM personal computer was introduced in 1981 and the Apple Macintosh in 1984. In 1982 *Time* magazine declared the computer "man of the year". By 1986 the number of computers in the United States had risen to over 30 million, jumping to 50 million in 1989, the year that the first notebook computer appeared. In the same year, an academic billboard, called World Wide Web, was invented by Tim Berners-Lee. The last decade has seen an explosion in accessible bandwidth around the world, allowing increasingly powerful and flexible computers to interact with each other in real time. In 1993 the first browsers were introduced, closely followed by the Internet, effectively giving public access to millions. Today there are over 5000 ISPs around the world that will service a projected 250 million email accounts for about 150 million Internet users per year. Traffic on the Internet doubles every 100 days. This stunning change in the way the world does business was totally unpredicted even five years ago.

Strengths and weaknesses of the Internet and email

These will be comprehensively covered in Chapters 7 and 8, as there are so many clinical issues of significance that are specific to the Internet, especially Internet addictions and phobias.

The Internet is fast gaining international acceptance. It is widespread and accessible, becoming cheaper, better understood and more user-friendly and flexible, with access by satellite to laptops and palm-sized computers, and even via videophones. On the downside, the Internet is overloaded and can be a great time waster. Remember to always "bookmark" your favorite sites so that you don't spend hours trying to find them the next time you log on.

Also guaranteed to raise your blood pressure is the Internet's tendency to suddenly drop out when it becomes overloaded. This can be particularly disturbing if you rely on email for your work. Many such people, myself included, maintain accounts with two different ISPs so as to guarantee access at all times. But perhaps the most annoying thing about the Internet is the way sites come and go. Sites are usually set up by individuals, and if they lose interest, don't pay their ISP dues, or simply change their address, the homepage suddenly disappears, usually without a hint as to whether it has moved or died completely. For this reason it is always worth checking out any homepage to find out when the site began. Be wary of brand new sites that don't seem to have had much thought or effort put into them — they will probably be gone next month! But this weakness is also a strength, because the Internet is constantly changing and alive, and good sites are regularly updated to encourage return visits.

What evidence is there that e-health works?

Actually, not much! Given that most scientifically valid clinical research projects take six months to plan, six months to attract funding and resources, at least a year or more to complete and several months to analyse and write up results before the final wait for publication in a scientific journal, this is hardly surprising. Remember that the Internet is still in its infancy, so the usual research cycle of about three years from planning to publication of results has hardly had time to be completed. There are some early evaluations of psychotherapy by email that look positive, but otherwise the Internet is like the phone

— everyone just assumes it works but no-one has really proved it!

And one of the reasons there has been so little evaluation is the large number of disparate interest groups — all with their own agendas — who are involved in e-health.

The players

This is where it starts getting complicated. There are so many groups, each with a high opinion of its own worth and all looking for a bite of the cherry, their share of the profit. These stakeholders cover the gamut of health, education, information technology, finance, defence and social service industries. There are six main groups:

Patients and their families, doctors and other health professionals

Mostly these people are united and driven by the simple desire for better-quality health care. This is the most important group for e-health.

Teachers, researchers and students

These are the people who observe and evaluate the process of e-health. At present there aren't many of them, but they are extremely important because their research will demonstrate the effectiveness, or otherwise, of the online care. This research will ensure that the therapies are used properly and are funded in the future.

Governments, politicians, professional bodies and unions

This is the group that will regulate and attempt to control the development of e-health. They are also the major funders who need to be convinced of the efficacy of e-healthcare so it can play an even more central role in the provision of health services world-wide. Politicians love e-care systems — as long as they don't have to pay too much for them — because they offer huge possibilities for self-publicity and vote garnering.

Hardware and software developers and retailers

These vary from the profit-driven multinationals like Microsoft, Intel and Sun to idealistic individuals who develop software programs or useful clinical gadgets in their homes purely in the hope of helping someone. There wouldn't be any online services without these people, but beware the motivations and ruthlessness of the multinationals in particular. There have been many excellent ideas, systems and programs bought by large companies and deliberately sunk without trace to eliminate competition.

Telephone companies, carriers and Internet providers

These provide the basic infrastructure necessary to carry the online therapies and, again, they are driven by profit. Controlling access to the networks is of critical political importance and the struggle to control this access should not be underestimated.

Consultants, entrepreneurs and hangers-on

Occasionally these people are helpful. But more often than not, in my experience, they are out for short-term financial gains for themselves, usually at the expense of the users — the patients and clinicians. Beware the "consultant" with generic skills and little useful knowledge. Male versions wear dark suits, have greased-back hair and are permanently glued to mobile phones. The female version wears too much make-up, too few clothes and constantly flatters her potential employer. If they do win your contract, they will invariably recommend that further consultants (themselves) are employed to further the project in the next stage that they identify! They are drawn, like magpies, to any new and potentially lucrative area such as this, and are best treated with extreme caution and a healthy dose of cynicism.

The development of e-health involves collaboration between all these different groups. It must be remembered that online systems are simply part of an overall health system. They should not be seen as being ends in themselves but a means to broaden the choices of care available. As long as e-healthcare systems on the Internet are flexible, simple, have built-in training, are user friendly, are focused on patients' needs and encourage collaborative health efforts, they should be successful. Nobody said it would be easy!

CHAPTER 4
ONLINE CONSULTATIONS

There are a number of health options on the web for patients. All of these are available now in a variety of forms and will be discussed in this and the next two chapters. They include: information provision (for individuals or groups, general or personalised), diagnostic scales or instruments, health-risk calculators, support groups (chat lines or discussion groups, facilitated or not facilitated), expert interactive sessions, and email access to experts (known or unknown) for consultation.

Steps in the consultation process

Let's start with e-consultations. A consultation carried out online isn't very different from one you would have in a therapist's office or surgery. It might still incorporate:

- the referral process
- gathering information from the patient during the interview and from other people or sources before, during or after the interview
- assessing the patient's physical and mental state
- structured questionnaires and assessment tools
- feedback on the diagnosis and developing a treatment plan in consultation with the patient, relevant family members and the referrer.

Of course the success of these steps depends on the level of personal and professional trust and commitment between the patient and the doctor.

The referral process

Usually, the referrer sends information about the patient to the doctor. Increasingly people will self-refer on the Net to the doctor of their choice. Traditionally referral has been by letter, but increasingly it is being sent by email, and within a few years it will be sent by videomail. Patients will be video recorded during primary care consultations and the video emailed to the specialist along with any other essential information, such as EKG records and X-rays.

One of the benefits of e-health is that during this referral period patients will have the opportunity to find out about their doctor through the doctor's homepage or curriculum vitae on the "net". Of course, this is also a useful source of information for patients having face-to-face consultations.

Information gathering

Traditionally, information is gathered from the patient, the referrer and sometimes family and friends and other health-related services. Doctors need:

- basic demographic data — name, age, contact details, next of kin etc.
- history of present difficulties — symptoms, disability levels, length and extent of problems, previous attempts at treatment
- significant past medical, psychiatric and alcohol and drug use history, present medications and alcohol and drug intake
- family background and history — social and genetic
- personal history, including early development, schooling, relationships, work history and any childhood or other traumas.

The amount of information collected and the way in which it is collected varies enormously depending on the clinical situation and the requirements of the patient and the therapist. For instance, if I am doing an emergency face-to-face assessment I will often initially collect only information related to the first three points above. That may be all that is necessary or possible to collect in a stressful situation and will allow initial diagnostic and treatment decisions to be made.

All this information can be gathered either face-to-face or online (although the interview may take a little longer by email) or by phone if speed is of the essence. Structured interviews, either written or spoken, can be used to collect the required broad-based information, after which the doctor can then ask or email more specific questions.

Other sources of information, such as family, friends, carers or other health agencies, are contacted in exactly the same way with e-care as for face-to-face assessment. In both situations the patient should be informed of these contacts.

A word here on Internet therapists who don't insist on knowing the full name and contact details of their patients and who do not give out their own specific and correct contact details. These "therapists" should be viewed with caution. I do not consider that therapists, whatever their training, are acting professionally if they do not insist on knowing who their patients are. (Some organisations, such as the Samaritans, don't require contact details but they deal only with crises and don't treat people long term. This is different.)

Assessing the patient's physical and mental state

Most patients referred for e-health assessments should also have a physical check-up. If you are seeing your doctor face-to-face as well, and you use e-health for only some of your consultations, this is not a problem as any physical examinations required can be done in the normal way when you see your doctor in person.

But what if you are some distance from your doctor? It may seem a tall order to expect online doctors to make a diagnosis without a physical examination, but it's actually not. Experienced doctors base 85 per cent of their medical and psychiatric diagnoses on history alone, with no need for physical examinations, blood screens, Xrays etc. But there are, of course, many occasions when a physical examination is necessary. Well, the age of virtual physicals is almost with us. Several studies have shown that a nurse performing an examination for which he or she is trained, under the supervision of a doctor observing on a videosystem, is just as accurate at picking up physical abnormalities as the doctor in the live situation. However, video on the net is not always available, so the best alternative is to arrange for a local practitioner to do the examination and to tell them what to look for in particular.

Digital still or movie cameras are another possibility. These cameras can take pictures of skin lesions, abnormal movements, or close-ups of the eye and can then be sent as email attachments. In the same way X-rays, ultrasounds and pathology slides or results can be sent via the Internet from a patient or doctor to another doctor or hospital.

Assessing a patient's mental state is certainly more difficult online than face-to-face. Describing someone's mental state is the equivalent of a physician taking a patient's blood pressure. There are many different ways of describing a patient's mental state, but the following is the assessment guide I use:

- *Appearance* — the patient's physical presentation, clothing, hygiene and cultural appropriateness
- *Behaviour* — the patient's behavioural style, including agitation, slowness, or inappropriate or unusual behaviour
- *Conversation* — the content, including direct quotes, and the form of speech, including the rate and logic of the patient's thought processes
- *Mood* — the level and type of mood, its variability, range, appropriateness and intensity
- *Perceptual abnormalities* — symptoms of psychosis or other ab-

normal phenomena including hallucinations or delusions in any of the five senses of vision, hearing, smell, taste and touch

- *Cognition* — processes of orientation, memory, attention and concentration
- *Dangerousness* — suicidal or homicidal thoughts, beliefs or feelings
- *Insight* — what the patient believes is their problem, and how realistic this is
- *Judgment* — assessment of the level of judgment, particularly regarding decision making
- *Rapport* — the interaction between the patient and the therapist and, in particular, the feelings the patient evokes in the therapist.

This is actually just a simple way of describing anyone. Not all sections have to be completed. Sometimes it isn't possible to complete them all even in the face-to-face situation, but a large number of these questions can be answered using email.

There are ways around the problem of a lack of visual cues. Patients can provide photographs of themselves, have their relatives or friends give the therapist objective descriptions of them or they can fill out structured interview sheets which contain cognitive tests or questions about their symptoms.

On the other hand, a face-to-face assessment performed in the first instance makes phone and email follow-up much easier. The doctor and patient can get to know each other and the doctor will be more confident of his/her assessment of the patient.

The whole online assessment process will change dramatically with the introduction of videoconferencing on the net. The expertise that many doctors have developed through telemedicine will be transferred to the Internet and full online health assessments will become commonplace. These changes are not far away and will transform the face of health care.

Structured questionnaires and assessment tools

Most of us have filled out some sort of health assessment form at some stage of our lives. These are now widely used in all areas of health to help assess illnesses and disabilities as diverse as impotence, cardiac disease, schizophrenia and arthritis. Questionnaires are well suited to online assessments, to assist with diagnosis and to measure treatment outcomes. In my own clinic we use at least half a dozen different questionnaires. Some are very simple and some are long and complicated. Many of them appear on the Internet sites quoted in the appendix.

Patients can use questionnaires to monitor their own progress. One of my patients who has depression regularly uses the Beck Depression Scale to check his level of depression. When he comes to see me he brings his weekly rating results to help us measure his progress. Similar questionnaires are available for disorders such as asthma, pain, muscle and heart disorders and epilepsy.

Providing feedback on the diagnosis and developing a treatment plan

Following the assessment the patient should be given a full explanation of the diagnosis or problem. With email, the patient has the information in writing and can refer to it at a later date. And the doctor has a permanent record of exactly what has been "said" to the patient.

What consultations are available online?

Almost any consultations can be performed online! And an increasing number of practitioners are now performing them. Consultations fall into two broad groups — those performed by conventionally and professionally trained practitioners and those undertaken by "alternative practitioners".

Conventional clinical practitioners

These people are professionally trained in medicine, psychology, nursing or other professional disciplines. It is common for these groups to work in a multidisciplinary manner, each providing specialist input and expertise into the assessment and treatment of individuals with significant medical illnesses. A team approach based on the knowledge and training of individual professionals with overlapping and complementary skills can be very effective.

Patients who email me have usually seen me face-to-face previously, so my personal use of email for consultations is for follow-up rather than for intial consultations, or for when patients cannot get to see me face-to-face because I am overseas or in another state and they want an urgent response to a particular problem. As I know them already, I can almost always give them advice which saves them having to go to an unfamiliar doctor.

In crisis situations where time is critical telephones are the time-honoured solution. Patients with specific problems expect their doctor to help them quickly. To save time the doctor will spend less time exploring the patient's background and more time on the immediate problem and how to resolve it.

Crisis intervention by email can be between doctor and patient or between fellow sufferers, as in this example:

> Posted by Melancholy Guy. April 1999
> *Hey. I'm really at the end of my rope here. Need to hear three things 1. Is it worthwhile trying to keep on realising yourself when you're down? 2. Somebody out there must know what makes it worth living for. 3. Has real full-blown depression made me lose my centre. I'm dead and I'm not even thirty. What I'm depressed over*

is totally irrelevant to me. I'd rather have cancer than this. I look at people and I can't see their faces. I listen to them but I can't hear what they are saying. Will I ever hear and feel again? If not, what can I expect from life? I'm seeing a psychiatrist but he hasn't prescribed drugs yet. I can't tell him anything relevant about my life. I just feel dead. How can this all be. I'm not even thirty, and I've blown everything. Who can help me?

Reply by Lorna, shortly after:
Depression is a numbing event. I have my highs and lows. Luckily I have light in my life now. Frustration, no relationships, no job, failure — that's all part of being depressed and living in the social mayhem of the 90s. Whatever the case, have faith in your psychiatrist. A lot of things you mentioned sound like depression talking. You know that body chemistry and psychological aspects of depression are interrelated. If you feel bad physically, stress or something, don't take care of yourself, eat wrong, sleep wrong, and you can wind up feeling tired, irritable and depressed. You get a chem imbalance or something and feel bad physically. Whatever the reason, things will get better. I have been if far worse shape than I am now. I took antidepressants when I was like you. They won't "prove you wrong to yourself" but they can help you gain some perspective while you sort it all out. I am telling you this because #1 there is anonymity here #2 there is hope in this situation. Many many people feel like you do, and you will feel better someday. You will laugh again! Just keep seeing your Doc and don't give up! As you begin to feel better things around you will begin to look better.

Alternative practitioners

The most common alternative practices are hypnotherapy, yoga and acupuncture, and nutritional, orthomolecular, religious and spiritual therapies.

Many of these therapies are used for stress-related disorders and a large number are promoted as working on the mind–body interface. The Internet is a veritable gold-mine for those who are interested in alternative therapies, although, having waded through a large number of sites, many of very dubious quality, I could find none offering consultations by email. There are, however, a huge number of commercial sites selling everything from vitamins to light and sound machines to focus on your brain-waves! If you have a yearning to become "qualified" yourself, the Internet offers training in a bewildering array of therapies, often taking only a few days to complete and setting you back up to $1,500 a day.

The Yahoo site on alternative medicine (www.yahoo.com/Health/alternative_Medicine) contains links to a fascinating collection of subjects, such as:

- orthomolecular medicine
- naturopathy
- applied Kinesiology
- Chinese medicine
- homeopathy
- macrobiotics
- music therapy
- hypnotherapy
- meditation
- polarity therapy
- sensory deprivation
- biofeedback
- gemstone therapy
- iridology
- massage therapy
- breathwork
- yoga
- natural hygiene

If these all sound a bit tame, you can also link into the more unusual — such as "urine therapy" for those who fancy drinking their own urine or "trepanation" for those who believe that cutting a hole in the top of their skull is likely to let some light into their lives. I strongly advise against either of these delights!

As with all Internet therapies, be careful! Much of what is available is dubious in the extreme. Think hard before buying anything on these sorts of websites and consult with friends, family and conventional therapists before signing up for any expensive courses. At the very least, insist on seeing the qualifications and training experience of the therapists. Follow the recommendations in Chapter 6 on selecting an online therapist.

Important points to remember

- **It is essential that online assessment is as comprehensive as face-to-face assessment.** This should be possible in most online situations but does take more effort. It is crucial that your doctor or health professional has adequate and appropriate information in order to make correct decisions.
- **Information from a variety of sources is especially useful when working online and can usually be easily and rapidly obtained by phone, fax or email.** Some Internet sites have tremendous resources and links.
- **Many patients prefer the extra accessibility and choice that the e-health offers.** I have yet to meet a patient who hasn't wanted more information and choice about their therapeutic options. Gone are the days when the doctor or other therapist patronisingly taps you on the head and says, "There, there, don't worry, I know best" and makes all your health decisions for you.
- **If a therapist has any doubts at all about the effectiveness of a particular online consultation, he or she should always arrange a face-to-face one instead.** There is nothing clever about trying to use online technologies exclusively if a face-to-face consultation is possible and is preferred. This is especially so in an emergency or where someone has an acute illness.
- **Following the consultation, the doctor should provide written feedback to both the referrer and the patient.** I usually send the patient copies of the information I send to the referrer. Consultations are about information exchange and communication and the patient must be central to this process.

CHAPTER 5

TREATMENT AND PREVENTION ONLINE

An amazing fact is that two-thirds of the people who use the Internet use it for looking for medical information. And this involves 75 million people in the United States alone. The availability of good-quality health information on the Internet means that patients can find out more about their problems and sort out their own treatment options. Over the centuries, as we have radically changed our minds about the causes of illness, our ways of treating it have also changed. In 450 BC Hippocrates declared that melancholia was caused by excess black bile, and hysteria by a wandering uterus. Both these ideas remained influential into the 19th century! At other times in history, depression has been blamed on domination of the soul, gluttony, excessive masturbation, witchcraft, variations in the circulation of the blood, animal spirits and "bad humors". Fortunately treatments have also changed. We no longer burn people at the stake to destroy their inner demons as happened to many thousands of people in the 15th century.

Information-age health care

Dr Richard Smith, the editor of the *British Medical Journal*, has talked about the move away from what he called "industrial age medicine" to "information age healthcare". He looked at these two health systems in terms of the type of care provided and the cost. Smith showed how in the medicine of the past, and today, most costs borne by the community are for the actual health-care system itself, at primary, secondary and tertiary levels. Primary health care includes your primary care doctor and community services; secondary health care is the large number of hospitals around the world; tertiary care involves primarily the teaching hospitals in the major cities.

With information freely available, consumers having more power, and the technological and communications revolution, the move to information-age health care becomes both possible and, increasingly, a reality. Smith saw six levels of care for the future, and these are already emerging. Patients will increasingly be involved in individual self-care at the top and most important level, particularly in preventing the impact of illnesses. The second level of care involves patients' families and friends, while the third level is essentially networked self-care, such as is increasingly happening through self-help groups, many of which have a significant Internet presence. Professional care is eventually reached at the fourth level where clinicians, be they doctors or nurses, will act as facilitators or organisers of care, providing information and analysis of health information for patients to make their own health-care choices. The next level is physicians as partners in health care, in an equal relationship, working with patients to assist them in the treatment process. Only at the sixth level, where doctors are authorities, does one finally reach what is often thought of as being the traditional "doctor–patient relationship". Here patients turn to doctors for authoritative advice, and allow doctors to make decisions about their health-care choices. In future we will have to put more and more of our community resources into the levels of self and community care, and less proportionately into formalised health services.

Traditional health-care treatments fall broadly into three groups:

- biological and medically based
- educational, social and community-based therapies, interventions and prevention programs
- self-help and consumer support groups.

All these groups use the Internet — at present some more than others. But, as patients learn more about the Internet and health-care professionals become more flexible, the Internet will become increasingly important for assessment and treatment. But how can you efficiently find the right information about your health from that wonderful, disorganised, revolutionary medium that we know as the Internet?

Searching the Web — a rational strategy

It is certainly true that there is a great deal of misinformation on the Internet, and it is very hard to work out what is good and what is not. Most people who bring information to me that they have derived from the Internet tend to have far too much, literally bundles of print-outs, and much of it is poor quality. Interestingly, more than half of the searches for health information on the Web are being performed by partners, carers and loved ones of a sick person, and the single most common reason for Internet searching given by such people is that they are looking for information following the diagnosis of an illness in a loved one. The Internet can be excellent for finding useful information, but you need a sensible search strategy, especially when you are looking for accurate and specific information that will help you make rational decisions, rather than just surfing for fun. The following four steps are recommended as your Internet search strategy, whether you wish to find out what your doctor has published or what range of treatments are available for a particular illness. (Remember to look at the appendix for details of a wider range of sites than given here.) If you are not sure how to use the Internet or to perform searches, do the interactive tutorial course at http://www.netskills.ac.uk/TONIC

Professional journal searching

There are several free programs on the Internet which will allow you to search professional scientific papers from the health and medical journals. You might as well learn to search in the same way your doctor will. All of the scientific papers quoted in these databases will have been peer-reviewed. The two main professional databases are:

"Medline" (http://www.ncbi.nlm.nih.gov/PUBMED
"Psycinfo" (http://www.HealthGate.com/price/b.psycinfo.html)

Medline is a library search engine that reviews all important peer-reviewed medical journals. This is almost always where your doctor will look first. That a journal is "peer-reviewed" is important: experts will often have suggested significant changes or improvements to an article before publication. Many peer-review journals publish only 15 to 20 per cent of the papers they receive, so their standard is extremely high. At present Medline has 9.5 million citations with approximately 31,000 more added each month.

Psycinfo is published by the American Psychological Association and is the premier psychological database search engine. It is not as large as Medline but still covers the scientific contents of over 1300 journals in 25 different languages.

Getting the information you need from both Medline and Psycinfo is easy. First put in the topic of your search, for example arthritis. The search engine then gives you the number of papers that contain that word — in this case far too many! If you wish to make the search more specific, add extra keywords which will reduce the number of papers you get. Generally, it is best to start with a broad general word such as "arthritis" and then narrow down the search by following it with words such as "treatment", "males" and "outcomes". You would then get copies of all papers related to the treatment outcome of arthritis for males.

To obtain the background on your therapist, make sure you search on different variations of their name to find all their publications. For example, my scientific papers have been published under "Peter Yellowlees", "PM Yellowlees" and "P Yellowlees" and search engines won't discriminate between these different versions of the same name. If you just put "Yellowlees" into the engine, you will find all of my papers, but also a surprising number of other papers from other members of my family, and some people with the same unusual name that I have only heard of through the Internet!

Evaluated Internet subject gateways

There are a number of health sites that have been specifically set up to provide high-quality health information for patients and professionals; in the jargon of the Internet these are called "evaluated gateways". These sites attempt to ensure quality information by either using their own experts or linking only with other sites whose information they have carefully assessed or who have an acknowledged level of expertise in the area; major university sites are an example. They are also generally independent and run either by government agencies or consumer organisations; they do not take paid advertisments, and have effective quality mechanisms in place to ensure that biased information is less likely to occur.

The beauty of Internet searches is that you can pick up useful reliable information which hasn't been published in peer-reviewed journals. The gateways I use are the United States National Library of Medicine (http://www.nlm.nih.gov/

locatorplus/) or Healthfinder (http://www.healthfinder.org) in the United States, or OMNI (http://omni.ac.uk) or NHSDirect (http://www.nhsdirect.nhs.uk) in the United Kingdom. Other sites offer ways of evaluating the quality of patient information (http://www.discern.org.uk), and some are devoted to collecting peer-reviewed "best practice" treatment guidelines (http://www.guideline.gov) which you can use for comparison with your own treatment regime. If your therapist doesn't know about these sites, please tell them. If you want information on evidence-based medicine, you cannot go past the Cochrane Library (http://www.update-software.com/cochrane.htm).

One site we will hear a lot more about in the future is http://www.gomez.com. Gomez is a massive site that is dedicated to attempting to objectively rate and assess other websites on specific quality criteria. At present Gomez has rated over 20,000 sites and in recent times has started a rating process for health sites. This is the only site I have found that gives a "league table" of the many commerical sites, and in particular of those sites that offer interactive real-time question and answer email sessions with qualified doctors. If you want to put a quick question to an online doctor, this is probably the best place to access a list of available practitioners.

You may prefer to go to the gateways before doing a database Medline search, because these are still reliable sources, and tend to have more systematically presented information that often summarises areas of interest, whereas Medline picks mainly scientific papers which are usually much narrower in their content. Take your pick.

Web searches

With the Web you will need to question the quality of the information you retrieve much more critically, as most of it will not have been subjected to any quality review mechanism, and much will have a commercial bias. There are numerous search engines on the Web, and they all serve the same function. They attempt to find as much specific information as you request, as easily as possible. But of course they are all different, use different search approaches, and cover different sets of sites.

I mainly use three such engines when looking for health-related information for patients. Alta Vista (http://www.altavista.com) is huge and indexes over 150 million pages, but it has quite a good advanced engine which can make your search more specific. Yahoo (http://www.yahoo.com) has a good health search engine, with a particular emphasis on consumer information, and a well set out strategy for defining your question more accurately. Perhaps the most comprehensive is Google (www.google.com) which is a fascinating engine with quite good linked search strategies, but with the ability to prioritise websites that receive the heaviest traffic, hence you receive the most popular sites first. There are several more sites listed in the appendix, and you can always go to the various commercial health portals, whose main strength is their immediacy and their ability to bring you up-to-date health information from all sorts of sources. Consider also subscribing to their electronic newspapers, especially if they can send you only news stories that match search criteria that you have defined.

Research by Tom Ferguson (1998) on patient requirements of the Internet has shown that one of the main needs is for good "frequently asked questions" responses. Most health sites have these, but one site, http://www.FAQ's.org, has amalgamated frequently asked questions by disease, so that it acts as a single source of patient-focused information in this area.

Try doing some Internet searches on your online or face-to-face doctors, as the information you'll find on the Internet will probably be very different from what you glean from a journal search. The Internet search may turn up some of the same academic papers, but you may also find your doctors on other websites — maybe they play in a rock group or on a sports team. They might have their own website and their curriculum vitae might be available online. All this information will give them a human face and help you to decide whether they are right for you.

If your online doctor or practitioner does not have any Internet presence, the alarm bells should be sounding, because they should at least be providing basic information about themselves for you to check.

Discussion lists and newsgroups

The final part of your strategy is the one where you can waste the most time, and where the information is least reliable. But it can be fun and is sometimes helpful. You might be lucky and join a group where there is a real expert who can answer your precise questions. Increasingly these "expert mediated" chat forums are being advertised on the Web, and judging by the number of commercial sites that offer them, they must be popular. To find these groups go to either DejaNews (http://www.dejanews.com) or Listz (http://www.listz.com/), where you can browse astonishing volumes of lists and decide if you want to join. If you have a very specific question that is somewhat unusual, it is well worth "putting out the word" to relevant lists — you will hit gold surprisingly often. In your bookshop, or online retailer, it is not too difficult to find books that have been written describing multiple lists and discussion groups as well. (In the area of mental health, Dr John Grohol's book *The Insider's Guide to Mental Health Resources Online* (1999) is an excellent example.)

Do be careful with discussion lists and chat rooms. There

are some very misleading people out there, and I know of examples where patients have been put off having the best medical treatment available, particularly for cancer, because they have been given wrong or potentially dangerous information in a chat room. Dr Gary Doolittle (personal communication, 2000), an excellent oncologist from Kansas with years of experience in telemedicine, who also encourages his patients to email him, has seen this happen on several occasions, and has had to spend quite a lot of time providing accurate information to previously misinformed patients so that they can make the best choice about their cancer therapy. Treat the information you get in chat rooms with the same degree of critical scepticism as you would of information gained in a casual conversation with people you have only just met at a social function.

Now that you know how to search the Internet in a rational and organised manner, let's look at the types of treatments on offer.

Biological and medically based therapies

Most illnesses have a basic biological cause, often genetically related, and may be triggered by physical or psychogical stress. Stresses include psychological traumas such as rape, social distress such as unemployment, and physical stress caused by accidents, head injuries and alcohol or drug abuse. Most illnesses are treated with a combination of medications as well as by educating patients and their families.

Both approaches to treatment may occur online. It is well known that doctors base 85–90 per cent of their diagnoses on a patient's history alone, so, as long as the doctor or therapist is able to make a good detailed assessment, treatment can be effectively carried out by telemedicine, email or phone. The following case study is an example of a combination of treatments using several technologies, practitioners and therapeutic modalities.

Joan is a 51-year-old farmer's wife living on an isolated property in Northern Australia. Her last child moved away to the city to find work, she suffered from chronic back pain from years of heavy lifting around the farm and she was often lonely. Her husband worked long hours on the farm and was constantly irritable, tired and worried about finances. The future looked bleak. None of the children wanted to take over the farm and a property slump meant that selling it was not an option. Joan was depressed and in constant pain.

The Royal Flying Doctor Service assessed Joan on telemedicine at her local bush clinic. She was diagnosed as having severe arthritis and major depression and was given an explanation of her disorders. Further information was provided through an Internet mental-health site run by a pain support group. The clinic nurse kept in close touch with her by phone and fax and made occasional visits, helping her with some simple cognitive techniques to improve her mood and cope better with her pain. The flying doctor saw her every fortnight, and her treatment program, involving regular painkillers and antidepressants, was overseen by a psychiatrist who reviewed her by telemedicine every couple of months, and who she was able to contact by email on a weekly basis. She gradually improved and after a year was taken off the antidepressants. She continued to keep in close contact with the clinic nurse who had become as much a friend as a therapist.

There are also online pharmacies on the Internet. It is possible for you to obtain a prescription from a doctor online, order your medication from the online pharmacy and even have it delivered to your door. But make sure that your doctor knows what you are doing and what medication you are taking! There are a lot of important practical and ethical issues involved here, and these will be dealt with in Chapters 7 and 8.

Multinational pharmaceutical companies are now dovetailing the release of new drugs with the formation of 24-hour telephone centres staffed by nurses to provide advice and information on these new drugs. The patient's doctor is also notified by fax or email of any inquiries from their patients so they can follow-up if necessary. It is inevitable that these companies will become more aggressive in the future, and will directly market to patients via the Internet — again raising many ethical and practical issues.

Educational, psychological, social and community-focused therapies and interventions and prevention programs

Prevention is always better than cure. There are many ways to prevent illness. These are mostly through community education and behavioural change, leading to more immunisations, better ante-natal care and better nutrition, for example. In the first ten to fifteen years of our lives we have the ability to soak up masses of information. This is when many of our lifelong habits are formed. Although there are some preventive health programs for young children and adolescents, most are poorly thought out, taught by non-experts and are often not easy to access. Sadly, knowledge about healthy relationships and lifestyles is mostly seen as less important than the traditional "3 Rs" — Reading, Riting and Rithmatic! We know that certain types of behaviours are risky and that some occupational groups tend to be more affected by certain disorders than others. Doctors are a good example. Many doctors abuse alcohol and drugs, have marriage problems and have a higher than average rate of suicide. They tend to be hard-working, focused individuals who often put work before outside interests. They manage their own stress badly while continuing to help others.

The sad thing is that although we know how to prevent many disorders, we have not done much about it. The advent of online technology is changing this and over the next few years will have an enormous impact in delivering prevention strategies.

How online technology will help prevent illness

Pregnant women can now be screened and their pregnancies monitored more effectively. If they or their children are at high genetic, social or medical risk they can be given special attention. The children can be followed-up more closely and comparisons can be made using case registers — large collections of data held online from similarly affected children — to detect any developmental abnormalities as soon as possible. Online education about healthy eating and exercise during pregnancy is available and many women are now monitored by both their obstetrician and their primary care physician in a process of "shared care" that increasingly requires the exchange and sharing of electronic medical information.

Mass education on health is needed to prevent illnesses and some countries are now getting serious about this. Malaysia has four e-health projects in the pipeline. One is a massive public health education program, with online outlets planned all over the country. Similarly, Singapore plans to make the Internet accessible to all citizens within the next few years and Korea is building a health-focused "cybercity".

The various talking therapies are, of course, ideal for the Internet. If you can provide psychotherapy by letter, as used to be the case, then it is certainly possible via the Internet, and even more so as the multiple communications technologies coalesce and become more powerful. Cognitive-behavioural psychotherapy, or CBT, is the "thinking and doing" approach to therapy. The cognitive, or "thinking", component assumes that we develop certain set patterns of thoughts which we then act on consciously or unconsciously. Hence if we think in negative patterns we get negative outcomes and will become depressed. The therapeutic task is to confront the negative thoughts and replace them with a more positive set to gradually relieve the depression. The "doing", or behavioural, component is like training an athlete to improve their performance: the anxious person who hyperventilates is taught to control their breathing and relax; the alcoholic is taught to reduce their drinking by avoiding stimuli that have led to drinking in the past; the asthmatic is taught to differentiate between shortness of breath caused by asthma and that caused by anxiety.

Internationally renowned British psychiatrist Professor Isaac Marks MD (1998) is heading a team which is developing self-treatment programs for patients with obsessive-compulsive (OCD) disorders. By reacting to cues given during a personal or computer-conducted telephone interview, patients could successfully assess their own condition at home. These patients were able to rate the severity of their OCD and depression, as well as monitor how much it was affecting their work and social lives.

On-line computer programs to treat many anxiety and phobic disorders are now available. Many still require a therapist to be present at least part of the time, but some, often designed like multimedia games, can be used by patients on their own. One example is *Fear Fighter*, developed in England for patients with agoraphobia and panic. In its first trial, 6 out of 15 patients improved "dramatically or moderately" in 12 computerised sessions without any therapist present.

The ultimate form of online CBT is "virtual reality therapy". By simply wrapping on your surround sound and vision multimedia headset you can be instantly transported to a cliff edge, soar in a plane thousands of feet above the ground or simply be surrounded by a gathering of thousands of spiders — depending on your phobia.

Using virtual reality technology patients with a fear of heights have been treated with integrated visual displays, body tracking and other sensory input devices in a computer-generated virtual environment. And these treatments are rapidly becoming more available. The next generation of virtual reality programs are being designed to treat post-traumatic stress disorders caused by wartime experiences. Rather than the traditional method of confronting old nightmares, online technology will be able to deliver treatment in a far more therapeutic and humane way. Patients will be "transported" to the battlefront and fears and traumas will be resolved in virtual place and real time.

At a more mundane level, important personal experiences of Internet psychotherapy are now becoming available. The following was published at www.metanoia.org:

> *I am fairly knowledgeable about psychotherapy (for a lay person) and was fortunate to work with a very talented psychotherapist for several years, experiencing the full depth and richness of that experience. I also had the experience of corresponding by email with another psychotherapist over a period of about six months. I experienced deep emotions while reading and writing — grief, anxiety, joy, love, rage, you name it — and explored some very deep issues. I learned to trust and depend on this person. The therapist was usually able to sense my feelings from changes in my writing. Transference happened. The relationship was reflected in my dreams. I was challenged, comforted and empowered. The experience was profoundly healing, and my life changed for the better.*

This description shows that it is possible to have a deep and therapeutic relationship by email. If we accept that the relationship or bond is the main healing factor in most dynamic psychotherapies, then psychotherapy by email must be possible. The increasing numbers of people falling in love on the Internet is further proof that deep relationships are possible online. If you still doubt this, then think of books and literature — the power of the written word. Throughout history relationships have been maintained and enhanced through letter writing. Perhaps it has happened to you. Think of the authors that you love, whose writing styles you adore. Even though you've never met them you form relationships with them through their books.

Even group therapy is available on the Internet. Yvette Colon, an experienced social worker, has facilitated two therapeutic groups in an online community called Echo (www.echonyc.com/~women/Issue17/public-colon.html). It has given her a fascinating insight into the dynamics of group therapy online.

> *Online groups, depending on how they are structured, can offer an immediate feeling of safety that makes members feel comfortable. This can allow members to achieve closeness at a safe distance, resulting in their feeling less inhibited to examine aspects of themselves or issues that they might hesitate to explore in a face-to-face group. Increased self-disclosure and bonding can occur earlier in the online group process than in a traditional group, and this blurs marks of difference like race, culture and sexuality.*

It will be fascinating to see where online dynamic psychotherapy leads. Dr Ellen Rothchild notes that

> *psychotherapy by letter is nothing new; Freud analysed "Little Hans" this way. He also conducted his own self-analysis with*

Fliess by letter. Perhaps it's a shame that Freud is no longer alive — he would have loved the opportunity to use online technologies!

Having said all this it is important to remember that psychotherapy by email is more difficult, may take longer and is not generally preferred if it is possible for you to see your doctor face-to-face. Online psychotherapy is generally more tiring for therapists than face-to-face. Talking to a screen or typing solidly for several hours to a series of patients is more strenuous than seeing patients in the office. And it is not much fun staring at a computer or TV screen all day!

Self-help and consumer-focused groups and therapies

The Internet is home to an extraordinary number and variety of online groups and self-help or support programs, many owned and run by patients for their own special needs. Some groups are obviously therapeutic, sometimes set up or mediated by health professionals. They exist as mailing lists or news groups, where meetings are spread over periods of days — asynchronous meetings. Or they may be real-time conferences or chats using synchronous communication. The single main advantage of "cyberspace" for patients and therapists is that people with similar interests and concerns can meet each other easily.

The following was posted by Andrea in response to a question about what was good and bad about online groups (September 1998).

I like the online forum because it gives us the chance to talk things through without hurting friends or family. If I said some of the things I have said here to my boyfriend, for example, I know he would misinterpret me and not be objective. Here I can get some support from people who just want to help rather than because they have an ulterior motive in seeing me act in a certain way. Sometimes we just need someone to listen and if we give out to those around us it makes them really upset or angry. If I rabbit on and on here then I feel no one is going to reply to me unless they really want to. It helps me a lot because I'm not troubled enough to be on meds or anything, but I do get depressive episodes which I find difficult to deal with. And sometimes we can really make someone feel better without even knowing their full name!!

People are finding that on the Internet there is always someone to listen and give support in a safe and anonymous environment. The following are some examples in a "net-shell":

On alcohol

May 1998. Posted by Dodo

SHIT!!! I've been grogging on for years to ease my anxiety. I'm in a vicious cycle — on a downward spiral. The alcohol doesn't work — it's just a temporary sedative that wears off. Your problems bounce back. I've drunk so much that I'm addicted to the f. stuff. I'm in danger. No f. doctor will give me any meds to dope me up. I'd rather take them than booze. Anyone else the same?

Reply by Cas

I'm 33 and have been addicted to alcohol for 20 years. I quit drinking 3 years ago but started up again a year ago. It was the most foolish thing I ever did. When I was in my 20s I played in a traveling rock band and drank so much (constantly) I was having DTs by the time I was 26 (convulsions — audio/visual hallucinations, delerium). I also have had panics and anxiety for about as long as the booze which always made it worse (when I started drinking the next morning which I usually did). To cut a long story short I quit drinking for good on April 30th and will never drink again for as long as I live. I take more pills than my shrink likes but now take them to feel normal, not to be cooked. I used info at a website to keep me rational and will send details.

On obesity

Posted by Obscene. June 1999

Does anyone else eat and eat, continuing to destroy themselves? At 253 pounds I wake up every morning and say "this is the day I will do it!!". And every day I fail. Every day I look in the mirror and I am stunned at how much weight I have gained. Sometimes I don't even recognise myself. I hate the way I look and yet I love the comfort of food. I'm terrified of feeling hungry. I wish I could unzip some great zipper and step out of my fat self. Tonight has been especially bad — I have eaten soooo much. I feel so sad, alone and fat.

Reply by Jennifer

Yes! I always loved my food, but had been keeping things mostly under control until my older daughter committed suicide in June 1995. After that I seriously overdid it on food, and ended up gaining 60 pounds (and I'm short so it looks a lot more). I am currently battling with Food Problem by switching to lower-fat foods and exercising almost every day. The weight is coming off slowly. I've also got help getting over my daughter's death and that has helped me control my urge to eat whenever I feel sad. Try making small practical goals, like "today I will walk around the block" instead of "from this moment on I will be perfect".

Reply by Carrie

I had to mail you right away because I know exactly how you feel. I used to weigh 210 pounds and loved chocolate. Do females buy more chocolate than males? I've found out that there are no bad foods — you just have to modify the amount. I still eat chocolate and ice cream, but now I am addicted to exercise rather than food. It was difficult changing and I only started with walking half an hour three times per week. I now walk the dog for an hour each day, do weights three times per week, biking, aerobics and roller-

blading. It's all possible. Hang in there and keep some positive thoughts — I know you can do it.

While these examples are uplifting, as in everything there are potential downsides, and in the case of the Internet one of these is junk email.

Dealing with junk email

Junk email is a real curse. As a doctor who practises e-health I receive chain letters, invitations to pornographic sites and direct pitches for various products. It's a real problem for people whose email address is widely known. It is intrusive and personally disturbing. This is cyberspamming.

The speed and ease of email means that literally hundreds of thousands of direct mailings can be sent at the touch of a button. Recipients of these unsolicited mailings can feel vulnerable and exposed. Who knows your address? How did they get it? Who is it being passed on to? How will they use it? What is going to turn up in the email next?

Each time you log on to a chatline, to a newsgroup, or even to some homepages, your personal email address can be grabbed. Your rights to privacy are endangered as your address is added to thousands of others, and then unscrupulously sold to companies with the ethical principles of a sewer-rat in a cesspit. It's estimated that spammers reap US$0.003c for each filched email address they sell to commercial "sales" lists — that's US$300 for every 10 million addresses. It is so cheap that it's hardly surprising we receive uninvited junk email!

So what can you do about it? First, most good Internet Service Providers have filters which they set to cut out well known, or notorious, spammers. There are some other simple options that you can use to minimise the amount of junk email that comes in, and to deal with it when it arrives. Dr Martin Van

Der Weyden (1998), editor of the *Medical Journal of Australia*, suggests that you think before sending messages to news groups or giving personal details to a website, subscribe cautiously to discussion groups, and use your email program's filtering system. Some people use several email addresses, keeping separate addresses for personal and business matters.

But what to do when the junk email starts arriving? A colleague of mine, who had been a member of an anti-cult discussion group, suddenly started getting hundreds of messages per day from cults all over the world. They had obtained his address and were determined to stop his right to privacy and free speech. Another friend became so desperate he changed his email address and started all over again, which was most inconvenient. My personal solution is to read the name of the person who is sending the message and the message title. If neither ring any bells, I simply delete the message unread. If it was a genuine message I know that the sender will phone me or try again. And that's a great way of avoiding viruses like the "love bug".

I advise you to go carefully. There are many Internet sites recommended throughout this book and in the appendix. Log on to the Internet and visit the sites that interest you. You will learn lots. Go for it sensibly — and good luck!

CHAPTER 6

HOW TO CHOOSE AN ONLINE DOCTOR OR THERAPIST

Doctors and therapists on the Internet vary from the very bad to the excellent with many in between. So how do you choose a good one? I can see you throwing up your hands in horror, but read on — you *can* sort out a doctor who is right for you! It will take a bit of research, but it's better than taking short-cuts and maybe ending up with the wrong person. Ideally, of course, your Internet doctor will be the same doctor you see face-to-face, so you will know each other in both environments, and make a choice as to whether you have your consultations live or in cyberspace, at home or in the surgery, or even by the pool.

Dr Tom Ferguson (1998) has classified doctors consultation styles on the Internet into two types. He talks about Type 1 doctors who are "advisors, coaches and information providers" but who specifically do not attempt to diagnose or treat. These doctors, or other health professionals, are typically available through their own sites, or through the many commercial sites. They generally don't advise the same patient twice, and usually don't even give their name (although the commercial sites "guarantee" that they are fully qualified), and will often refer you to a local face-to-face doctor or hospital. Interestingly, this is how many of them receive payment for their services — the sites get a "spotter's fee" from local services that they refer people to. So there is an immediate conflict of interest and potential pressure on the type 1 doctors to refer people only to particular local health providers who have agreed to pay this fee. The best single place to find these medical advisors is through the league table of commercial sites at http://www.gomez.com. I am not recommending any particular doctors from these sites because it is impossible to tell how good they are.

Type 2 doctors are the majority of medical providers on the Internet. These are doctors like myself who provide normal face-to-face care, and who encourage their patients to also use email to contact them directly, which, as long as the guidelines for Internet consultations discussed in this book are followed, is a great way of working for both patient and doctor.

There is another group of health-care providers, however, who attempt to provide full health services only on the Internet. Many of these provide counselling or therapy services for mental-health problems, or alternative therapies of an often bizarre and inappropriate nature. At present my advice is generally to stay away from these therapists, unless you can be sure who they are and ideally can also see them face-to-face.

Full-time Internet health services and providers will become much more common in the next few years, and I predict that as many as 20–30 per cent of all health consultations will take place in cyberspace within 10 years or so. This will be a real revolution in health care.

Nowadays it's quite usual for patients to "check out" doctors and other health professionals before they visit them, but until recently it was hard to find out much mainly because of advertising restrictions. Patients had to depend on second-hand information and opinions. But times have changed. Several patients have come to me after reading my curriculum vitae on the University of Queensland website (www.coh.uq.edu.au). They chose me for my particular areas of expertise and skills, and made appointments directly with me rather than relying on their family doctor's referral.

Unfortunately, though, most people still fall upon their doctors by chance. Maybe you get a name from a friend, a neighbour or a chance acquaintance at the corner store. Maybe your doctor or health professional refers you, or an advertisement catches your eye. Sometimes you've no choice and you're referred through the health system. In future you'll be able to check out the credentials of your potential caregiver on the Internet, or even find a good doctor from scratch there. And this will apply whether you intend to see your doctor online or face-to-face, whether they have a particular speciality, or whether they live close by.

Internet therapy — a growth industry

Therapy is big business in the health world. Most family doctors spend about a third or more of their time helping people with stress-related problems, and there are a number of counsellors, psychologists and psychiatrists who see individuals for therapy as well. Using the Internet for counselling or psychotherapy is still in its infancy but it's expanding rapidly. Nobody knows just how many therapists work on it. One of the problems is that therapy goes under so many names: counselling, web-therapy, cybertherapy, online therapy, e-therapy, individualised information, individualised advice, behavioural telehealth, Internet health provision and Internet interactions, to name a few! When I recently put the word "counsellor" into the Alta Vista search engine it returned over 4 million mentions on websites, while the word "therapist" returned over 2 million pages.

Let's look first at practitioners who say they are specifically interested in mental health, and who provide paid services on the Internet. In May 1998 Terri Powell (1998) from the University of Kentucky sent out a questionnaire to the fifty online practitioners listed with the Metanoia website — currently the most comprehensive listing of mental-health practitioners. Only 13 of them replied, but in 1997 they "saw" a total of 1344 clients for an average of three times each. The year before, 8 therapists worked with 947 clients, and the year before that, 7 therapists worked with just 445 clients. In other words, this small group of practitioners doubled in size and tripled its number of clients in only two years! If it continues to grow at this rate, in ten years there will be 416 active counsellors registered on this one site alone, consulting with more than 300,000 patients. And this is actually a gross underestimate, as the survey was confined to America and the figures extrapolated from only 13 online therapists. Obviously Internet-based online therapy is set to be a massive world-wide industry.

A typical Internet therapist

In her study, Powell (1998) paints an interesting picture of what she called the composite Internet counsellor.

> *a 48 year old male psychologist with 15 years experience in traditional clinical practice. He's been in online practice for almost 2 years and calls his service, "advice giving". When you visit his website, you'll find that he uses some sort of encryption software to protect your anonymity. In order to reduce fraud and exploitation, his credentials have been authenticated. He believes that online mental health services increase clients' access to mental health professionals, especially clients living in remote areas or suffering from disabilities. The average client wants help with relationship problems or depression.*

General medical problems

Now let's look at other areas of health and see what Internet doctors are available for general medical problems. You can have almost any question you want answered by a type 1 doctor on the Internet, usually within a few minutes. But you have little idea of how experienced the doctor is who is answering you, and no recourse if the information is wrong. There is no overall reliable listing of doctors on the Internet, but they are not difficult to find. As stated earlier, use the search strategy from Chapter 5 and go to http://www.gomez.com to look at what I consider the best list of sites offering type 1 consultations online. Remember that the large commercial sites receive literally millions of hits per month, so they are unlikely to be able to provide personal service. If you want more than type 1 consults, particularly if you wish to receive the majority of your treatment via the Internet, I suggest that you search by your illness or need, in a structured way, and then ask the questions in this chapter. Names of doctors will often be found in chatrooms. Again go carefully and check them out. Dr Tom Ferguson has published an interesting list of his "top 10 tips" on cyberdocs on the Ferguson report at his website (http://www.fergusonreport.com). Have a look at that.

Do I want an online doctor?

Ideally you will have a doctor you can trust who you can choose to see face-to-face or online, depending on your choice and mutual convenience. But there are many situations where you will need to choose a specific doctor who you will consult online, and this will become increasingly common as health becomes a global industry. After all, why shouldn't you consult a doctor in Australia who is acknowledged as a world expert in say, liver disease, if your usual doctor in New York is uncertain as to your best treatment regime? (As well, the Australian doctor may be cheaper on the Internet than your own doctor because of the weakness of the Australian dollar in comparison to the US dollar!)

Look back through the descriptions in Chapter 2 of people who might benefit from e-healthcare. Do you fall into any of the categories? Maybe you simply prefer e-healthcare to face-to-face.

Check out your options. Speak to your doctor, go to the library, discuss your situation with your family, friends or partner and, if you are already seeing a doctor face to face, with them as well. You may decide to see an online doctor face to face for one session for a comprehensive diagnostic assessment, which should be conducted in a manner similar to that described in Chapter 4, before continuing to see them on the Internet afterwards. Alternatively, you may simply decide to do some surfing and access health information about your condition. Use the approaches recommended in this book in Chapter 5 and the sites suggested in the appendix.

If, by now, you believe e-health is right for you, it is time to look for an online doctor or health professional. You may have already found one in the course of your investigations, but I still suggest that you follow the guidelines in this chapter. Ask your doctor or therapist the questions in the second half of this chapter and be wary if they cannot, or will not, answer them. And don't forget to assess their website as well, perhaps using the tool available at the Discern website (www.discern.org.uk).

Face to face, or online?

If you are already seeing a face-to-face doctor but would like to consult an online health professional as well, explain this to your doctor, who needs to know so that mixed therapeutic messages do not occur that may not be in your best interest. Your usual doctor may also be able to give you the extra help you want. Don't give up on your face-to-face doctor too quickly. E-healthcare is still relatively new. We know that it can be effective, that it's an important adjunct to other treatment approaches, but until it is clearer in which areas it is most effective, it shouldn't be automatically assumed to be better than face-to-face care. In fact it's probably not in many instances.

To give you a feel for what's on offer from individual health professional sites, I have selected excerpts from some webpages which I have altered slightly to keep them anonymous. All these sites say that they employ professionally qualified clinicians with either medical, masters or PhD degrees. Some sound good and some not so good! You'll recognise why as we explore what to look out for later in this chapter.

Whether you need general guidance, are on the verge of a crisis, or are looking for competent peer review YYY may be able to help. We are not a substitute for face-to-face therapy, and may not be appropriate for everyone, but we do focus the attention of a group of highly skilled professionals on YOU! These are the same people who normally charge $100 to $200 per session! You need not send us your name, address or even phone number if you do not wish. All charges are discreetly billed to your credit card, and the therapist never sees your billing information.

XXX is the only Internet site that provides a LIVE physician-based interaction for patients in the comfort of their own home — a virtual housecall!! Whether at home, at school, or traveling within the country or abroad, XXX provides real-time, online, confidential consultative medical advice for our patients on the Internet.

My professional counseling rate is kept low, so you can afford it: just $90 per hour, charged to your credit card ... If you want to remain anonymous, it is not necessary to tell me your real name, even though you use a credit card. I understand that the issues you need to deal with may be nearly impossible for you to be open about under your actual name. So if you prefer, give me an alternate "working" name. I genuinely look forward to hearing *from you, to getting to know you and understand you. To gently exploring your areas of difficulty and pain. To achieving what none of us can do alone.*

Welcome to the first 24 hour telephone and online counseling service. There is no subject that is taboo. Whether you situation deals with sex, a relationship, gender issues, a past or present trauma in your life, substance abuse or addictions, eating disorders, a problem at work or home, depression, anxiety, phobias, parenting, an illness or just about anything else, we are here for you. All our counselors are licensed professionals (with Masters or PhD degrees) who care deeply about their clients and who work very hard to help them achieve the good health and peace of mind they desire in their lives. That's our goal.

Whichever treatment or online assessment and consultation you are considering, you should get a description of the philosophy behind the practitioner's approach, what type of consultation you are being offered and how long will it take. Ask these questions at the very beginning.

Obviously the doctor will have to perform a detailed assessment of your situation before being able to answer such questions. This assessment, in most clinical situations, normally takes at least an hour and may involve you filling in questionnaires and/or taking some tests. If you do not receive such an assessment, either by email, phone, face-to-face or even by videoconference, forget that health professional! How can they possibly know how to help you if they haven't taken the trouble to find out about you?

People choose their doctors with several factors in mind. Many people choose by gender — females, in particular, often prefer to see a female doctor. We also look at the doctor's expertise or experience with our problem. But, most commonly, we choose by price or availability — not a great way to guarantee a successful doctor/patient relationship! You wouldn't choose a car without checking it out, nor should you choose a doctor that way, particularly when you are in the modern-day equivalent of the wild west — the World Wide Web.

Assessing your e-doctor — ten questions to ask

You know now how *not* to choose a doctor, but how *do* you find the right one? There are ten questions you should ask. We'll look at each of the questions then work through how a good online doctor should respond. Remember to be friendly, businesslike, and don't take "no" for an answer. You are paying for the consultation. You are the customer. You must be satisfied with both the consultation and the consultant. These rules apply equally for an online or face-to-face health professional. Here are the questions:

- What are your qualifications and credentials?
- What experience do you have in offering face-to-face advice and e-care?
- Are you registered to practise in your own state or country and mine. Do you have appropriate malpractice insurance?
- Do you adhere to a documented code of ethics? Which one?
- What clinical and administrative guidelines for practice do you use?
- What areas do you have expertise in, and what evidence in the form of professional recognition, publications or lectures do you have to confirm this?
- Do you communicate with colleagues for professional supervision and self-development?
- Do you provide face-to-face support for your online patients if required?
- What are your billing procedures?
- Do you record consultations electronically in any way and, if so,

what are your consent and confidentiality procedures for this? How do you keep your clinical records, both face-to-face and online?

What are your qualifications and credentials?

No professional or ethical health professional from any background should mind being asked about their qualifications. They should be proud of their achievements. Indeed many doctors in office practice hang their qualification certificates in their rooms so that patients can examine them. Generally you should ensure that your e-consultant has either a medical degree or a masters level qualification in another relevant health profession. Sites such as http://www.doctorglobal.com include detailed biographies of the doctors who practise through the site and you should always check these details at any site you are using before consulting with any doctor on the Web. I am personally very wary of sites who simply say that they offer consultations by qualified doctors but do not give out the names and details of these physicians. Would you consult a doctor in the face-to-face world if you did not even know their name, never mind what their qualifications are?

The bottom line is that doctors offering e-care should have their credentials on a website. At the very least the site should contain details of their professional degrees and qualifications. It should also have a curriculum vitae showing academic and professional training, courses attended, special interests and expertise and any research papers or scientific publications they've contributed to. If they advertise a particular expertise, there should be evidence to support this, such as higher training or teaching and research skills. Doctors should always be prepared to answer questions about their credentials and their contact details should be found on the webpage. It's also good to find their photo. Photos contain lots of extra, often subconscious, information. The website may also contain links to the relevant pages of their professional organisation where you should find the relevant ethical guidelines.

I believe that it won't be too long before professional associations develop licensing for online practitioners. This will mean, for example, that the American Psychiatric Association will be able to tell you which psychiatrists meet the ethical and clinical requirements that the Association develops for e-therapies. The same will be true for the British and Australian Medical Associations and other professional bodies for both specialist and generalist practitioners. It will make the search for reputable e-practitioners much easier.

There are very few good credential checks available for doctors on the Internet. A site to start a credentials check for a mental-health practioner is www.metanoia.org. Here, "independent" reviewers rate online therapists' websites. The guide offers information about therapists' fees, credentials, services offered and confidentiality. Unfortunately, it doesn't assess the quality of the therapist's advice or counselling. Nevertheless, it's a good place to start and gives some ideas about how to check out other practitioners.

It is obviously not easy for patients to decide whether someone with a Masters degree in education is an expert in asthma advice and management, or whether a PhD in research methods equips a person to practise online hypnotherapy! Health practitioners come from many different backgrounds and unfortunately in many cases their training is non-existent or, perhaps worse, biased by their own philosophies or perspectives on life. Or they may simply be frauds.

My advice is that if an online health practitioner from any discipline is not registered with a professional organisation, don't go near them! Ask for their registration number so you can independently contact that professional body to confirm their membership. And do that.

What experience do you have in face-to-face health care?

An online practitioner must already be a very experienced face-to-face professional. Online consultations are more demanding than face-to-face ones. There are more potential pitfalls and greater organisational and ethical traps for the unwary. Except in exceptional circumstances, I don't believe anyone should offer online consultations without at least five years full-time face-to-face health experience. Don't be persuaded into seeing someone who is clinically inexperienced. Ask them about it. If they can't prove their experience, move on. It doesn't happen yet, but in future online doctors might have to provide testimonies of their skills from previously treated patients, just as happens when you choose a builder or architect.

Most online clinicians of the future will have secure websites where they will describe their skills and experience, communicate with patients and market their services. To check the quality of their site and the experience of the doctor, go through the following checklist:

1. Who is the author of the site? Perform a Medline or Psychinfo search as detailed later in this chapter to check out both the site author and the doctor. Frequently they are the same person.
2. Which institution supports the doctor and what affiliations do they have? Do they have an MD from Harvard as opposed to a diploma from the Dreamtime University of La-La Land?
3. Are the author and the doctor identified and can they be contacted? Avoid all health websites that don't have some sort of feedback or quality-control mechanism. And give them your feedback whether you like them, and the site, or not.

4. Is the information on the website current? Check out when the site was last updated (this is usually at the bottom of the homepage) and how often this occurs.
5. Is the information on the website balanced? I have yet to find a health-care issue with only one side to an argument or piece of advice. Even if the evidence for one particular approach is overwhelming, there will always be people who disagree and they should be represented or at least mentioned. Reputable sites will discuss possible biases, and will also declare any possible interests, particularly sponsorship-related conflicts of interest.
6. Can you verify the information on the website — particularly via hotlinks to other unrelated sites which are managed by different groups of people or organisations? Links to public libraries, universities and government agencies suggest better-quality information than links to commercial organisations, unusual religious sects or political parties!

Most importantly, find out if the website is trying to sell you something? Many health sites are linked to expensive "natural products" and the site is really no more than a shopfront for them. You should be skeptical about websites that have significant commercial sponsorship or advertising.

In general, look for sites displaying the logo saying that the site is set up according to the principles of the Health on the Net Foundation (http://www.hon.ch/HON/Conduct.html). These principles, quoted exactly from the site, are as follows:

Authority

1. Any medical or health advice provided and hosted on this site will only be given by medically trained and qualified professionals unless a clear statement is made that a piece of advice offered is from a non-medically qualified individual or organisation.

Complementarity

2. The information provided on this site is designed to support, not

replace, the relationship that exists between a patient/site visitor and his/her existing physician.

Confidentiality

3. Confidentiality of data relating to individual patients and visitors to a medical/health Web site, including their identity, is respected by this Web site. The Web site owners undertake to honour or exceed the legal requirements of medical/health information privacy that apply in the country and state where the Web site and mirror sites are located.

Attribution

4. Where appropriate, information contained on this site will be supported by clear references to source data and, where possible, have specific HTML links to that data. The date when a clinical page was last modified will be clearly displayed (e.g. at the bottom of the page).

Justifiability

5. Any claims relating to the benefits/performance of a specific treatment, commercial product or service will be supported by appropriate, balanced evidence in the manner outlined above in Principle 4.

Transparency of authorship

6. The designers of this Web site will seek to provide information in the clearest possible manner and provide contact addresses for visitors that seek further information or support. The Webmaster will display his/her E-mail address clearly throughout the Web site.

Transparency of sponsorship

7. Support for this Web site will be clearly identified, including the identities of commercial and non-commercial organisations that have contributed funding, services or material for the site.

Honesty in advertising & editorial policy

8. If advertising is a source of funding it will be clearly stated. A

brief description of the advertising policy adopted by the Web site owners will be displayed on the site. Advertising and other promotional material will be presented to viewers in a manner and context that facilitates differentiation between it and the original material created by the institution operating the site.

At www.mentalhealth.com Dr Phillip Long, the psychiatrist editor of *Internet Mental Health*, shows how to spot websites that depend heavily on corporate sponsorship. In one of his examples a sponsor's pharmaceutical product is mentioned 31 times with no references to any rival medications. A recent article in the *Washington Post* exposed the hidden link between a major health insurer and a very popular health portal which advertises itself as "The Trusted Source". Odd how such a trusted source couldn't tell consumers who owned it!

In reality sponsorship of websites is probably here to stay and it's likely that some popular sites will be heavily sponsored by unrelated products. Search engines, computer companies and www.Amazon.com, the huge online bookstore, already advertise on some health sites and, as long as there is no unhealthy conflict of interest, this should be encouraged.

Disclaimers are found on most health websites. Many online practitioners state that they are providing information, not giving proper health services, and are not to blame if the information is wrong or irrelevant. A fairly typical disclaimer on a site offering health information, discussion groups and chat lists, but not attempting to provide online consultations, reads like this:

The diagnosis and treatment of disease requires trained medical professionals. The information provided below is to be used for educational purposes only. It should NOT be used as a substitute for seeking professional care.

What experience do you have in e-care?

Don't forget to ask your potential e-doctor how many patients with your particular problem they have treated. Find out how those patients responded to the treatment, and what the consultant would do if you are one of the unlucky ones who doesn't recover in the expected manner. The answer to these questions is crucial. In future they should be on your doctors' website. At present, if you are not happy with the answer, move on to the next doctor.

Are you registered to practise in your state or country and mine? Do you have malpractice insurance?

All reputable online practitioners will be registered with a health licensing board, professional indemnity insurance company or professional association. Most will be with all three. You should arm yourself with your doctor's registration number and contact the associations to confirm that he or she is legally registered to practise. In the United States many registration bodies only allow doctors to practise in one state. Elsewhere it is more common for doctors to be registered to practise throughout their country. Make sure your practitioner is registered to practise not only in their country but in your country as well. International registration is cowboy country! In the future, global medical registration is inevitable, but currently all that doctors can do is register in all countries where they practise. This can be extremely difficult because of the different registration systems, standards and laws.

In some parts of the United States the potential legal ramifications of e-care malpractice are causing considerable disquiet. Luckily this doesn't appear to be such a problem in other countries where suing one's doctor isn't such a popular pastime. For patients, though, the bottom line is to make sure that your therapist carries appropriate malpractice insurance cover. Otherwise you have no comeback if things go wrong.

What code of ethics do you work by?

It is vital, and essential, that your online health practitioner adheres to a code of ethics — a set of rules and principles that govern the way they practise. If they belong to a professional body they will use that body's code of ethics which you should be able to read on their webpage. Basically, ethical rules state that a practitioner should never have a sexual relationship with a patient, that they should maintain confidentiality of patient records, and that they should provide treatment of the highest possible standard according to their knowledge and training.

What clinical and administrative guidelines do you use?

Most reputable online practitioners adapt treatment and administrative guidelines published by professional bodies to suit their own personal style, philosophy and skills. Check that yours does. The following are some examples:

Guidelines for email

The American Informatics Association recently published guidelines for doctors using email for clinical and administrative purposes. Among their recommendations are:

- Don't use email for urgent matters; use the phone or personal communications as you can't be sure when email will be answered.
- Ensure that patients know who reads your emails, how and where the emails are stored and whether copies are made and placed in your health-care notes.
- Decide with patients what type of transactions they should undertake using email, and define the type of transaction in the subject line of the message so that you can filter it quickly when reading

your email. Where possible use codes known only to you and the patient.

- Ensure that patients know that they should phone you or your consulting rooms if they don't get a response within an agreed period of time, say 48 hours.
- Agree not to forward possibly identifiable material about the patient to a third party without their express consent.
- Use encrypted email, if possible. This isn't always possible because encryption has to occur at both ends. If it is not practicable, ensure that the patient understands that the email is not secure.

Tele-homecare guidelines

Guidelines for patients receiving home care through telemedicine, videoconferencing using broad bandwidth, can be found on the American Telemedicine Association's website at http://atmeda.org. These guidelines are indicative of the sort of guidelines that will have to be introduced to e-healthcare on the Internet once videoconsultations are easily available over the Internet and real-time videoconsultations with your doctor become more common, especially from the home. Some of the more important points are:

For patients: "The first and last visit to the patient's home must be in person and not by video visit; patients may un-enrol from tele-homecare at any time; patients (or their caregivers) must be able to use and maintain the equipment and patients may not be viewed through the video without their knowledge or prior written consent."

For the treating person: "Personnel providing tele-homecare must document each video visit in the patient's chart; they may only make video visits within the limits of their expertise, a physician order must be obtained to integrate tele-homecare into the care plan, and, if 24-hour tele-homecare is not available, patients must be provided with written instructions for contacting after-hours care providers."

What are your areas of expertise? What evidence do you have in the form of professional recognition, publications or lectures?

Some health practitioners boast expertise in the most weird and wonderful things. Expertise in Projective Dynamism or Compulsive Dissociation sounds very important, but they are not recognised specialties! In fact I have just made both of these up, so beware!

Good doctors also teach; many carry out research. Increasingly doctors will have their qualifications, research references and teaching expertise detailed on their homepages but that is still relatively uncommon at present. There are other ways to check up, however; all you need to do is perform a literature or Internet search as described in Chapter 4.

Do you have access to colleagues for professional supervision and self-development? Can you access face-to-face support for your online patients if required?

Isolated doctors are potentially dangerous. Most health professionals have close ties with colleagues with whom they can discuss their most difficult patients for support and advice. Good practitioners realise that they don't know everything and are always seeking external reviews of their practice and opportunities to extend their learning. A potential downside of online health care is that doctors who spend much of their time online may not get the interaction with colleagues which is so important.

Your e-doctor must have a back-up system in place so that patients who are in severe crisis or are acutely unwell can receive immediate treatment and assistance in their own environment at any time. This is because most doctors only log on at certain times of the day and patients may have to wait 24 hours for a response to an email. This is obviously dangerously inadequate in emergency situations.

Legitimate email therapists, such as Martha Ainsworth at www.metanoia.org in the area of mental health, advise their patients what to do in an emergency:

> *If you are having suicidal thoughts you may need help immediately. Take yourself seriously. If your need is urgent, admit it. You deserve to get help, and to get it sooner rather than later. If you are experiencing intense emotional distress and need immediate response.*
>
> *Get off the computer and pick up the phone.*
>
> *Telephone a mental health hotline (numbers in your phone book).*
>
> *Otherwise call a psychotherapist, counseling centre or mental health clinic and make an appointment for an office visit. In urgent situations many therapists will see you on short notice. Be sure to make it clear that your need is urgent.*
>
> *SUICIDAL PERSONS MIGHT WISH TO READ THIS FIRST.*

This last message is in hypertext and links to some excellent advice from an anonymous patient aimed at persuading suicidal people to reconsider. This is therapy on the Internet at its best.

How do you bill?

Billing for online services has to be transparent and agreed to in advance of any consultations. Frauds abound on the Internet. Sadly common are the charlatans who set up non-secure websites then charge $20 to $50 per question on any health subject! You have no guarantee that the answer will be individual to you, has come from a particular therapist or is even correct! I have even found sites that won't give you any information about the site or the therapist unless you pay the question fee up front. The only thing you can guarantee is that they're happy to take your credit card through the only secure part of the site.

You are better to pay a well-qualified doctor by the hour to answer your questions, rather than pay by the question. Hourly costs vary from about $30 to $100. Not only will you get much better value, but your chance of getting the same practitioner for follow-ups is much greater.

When paying for health services with a credit card NEVER put your credit card number in ordinary email and NEVER use an unsecured website. Insist on using either traditional mail or bank transfer, a secure Internet payment service (your browser should tell you if it's secure) or fax or telephone your credit card number through to the doctor — making sure that the number you are ringing really does belong to the doctor. If your online practitioner rejects these options, assume it's a scam and don't pay.

Do you record any sessions electronically? If so, what are your consent and confidentiality procedures for this?

Confidentiality is crucial for any doctor, and even more so for the online practitioner. Fixed telephone lines are more secure than mobile phones. Ideally email messages should be encrypted, although this doesn't always happen. At the very least your doctor should check with you to ensure that you received his or her email, and should adhere to the email guidelines given earlier in this chapter. After all, emails do disappear into cyberspace, never to be seen again!

You must find out how your doctor keeps his or her clinical notes. How safe are these? Who else can access them? Most doctors using email simply print out and file their clinical emails into paper-based records at present. This is a far more accurate record than note-taking during a verbal exchange.

If you are not sure that your email messages are confidential, forget it. The following scenarios could make you think twice.

An employee receiving email counseling at his work address finds his email is being read (legally) by his boss. The embarrassed employee is fired and ends up more distressed than ever.

An explicit email from a patient to his doctor is accidentally sent to an entire email list of several thousand people, resulting in excruciatingly public humiliation.

A wife reads her husband's email in which he admits infidelity with other women and declares his love for his online doctor. She emails her husband and his doctor to acquaint them of her discovery, sends a copy of her husband's email to her lawyer, and changes the locks on the house.

By choosing the right online doctor you shouldn't end up in situations like these! Don't rush your choice, ask him or her the questions in this chapter and if you are satisfied with the answers you should be reasonably confident that you have found a professional e-healthcare practitioner.

Wrapping it up — bringing it all together

In short, the effective online doctor of the future will be:

- an experienced face-to-face doctor — competent and consumer focused
- able to understand, integrate and use a variety of information technologies, and also know when not to use them
- respectful of his or her patients and able to work with them in partnership
- trained in individual and group educational techniques
- an expert communicator with excellent media skills

- able to evaluate and analyse large amounts of health information, prioritise and provide best practice treatments
- constantly updating his or her skills and evaluating his or her own practice and the therapeutic outcomes of patients.

Find yourself someone who embodies all these ideals and you have found yourself the perfect online doctor.

CHAPTER 7

CHANGING RELATIONSHIPS

It doesn't seem very long ago (actually it was 1979) that as a raw young medical student I made my first ward round in an antiquated London hospital which, thankfully, no longer exists. The patients, terrified into submission by a ferocious senior nurse were laid out for the pleasure of the parading surgeon and his cortege of nurses and students. These patients were not allowed to speak as the surgeon made his pronouncements and decisions of great import, all the while tapping them patronisingly on the heads! The only expectation of the patients was that they look suitably grateful. If a patient had the audacity to question a decision, they were likely to labelled as noncompliant, a troublemaker, or having an "inadequate personality". I remember another student telling me that the only way to tell whether a patient on that ward was bleeding internally was to lift up the blankets at the bottom of the bed and see if the sheets were red! Thank heavens things have changed.

Today, patient–doctor relationships are much better. Online systems have exposed patients to a huge amount of health information, helping them to have an informed say in their own health care. This is balancing the scales of the patient–doctor relationship; medical paternalism will soon be consigned to the history books forever.

The therapeutic relationship

There are two components to the doctor–patient relationship: the empathetic component (how well the doctor understands you and tailors the treatment options to you as an individual) and the technical component (the expert knowledge which your doctor has learnt and uses for your betterment).

Professor Richard Wootton, who used to be Professor of Telemedicine at Queens University in Belfast, Northern Ireland, but who is now a colleague at the University of Queensland, believes that many people regard an excellent doctor–patient relationship as the gold standard in health-care delivery. Many patients today are dissatisfied with the traditional "Doctor knows best" attitude and Wootton believes that the emphasis on good communication in online relationships may mean that doctor–patient rapport will improve and regain its former high status. Clearly patients expect consultations to encompass both art and science. It is a fascinating paradox that a side effect of our technologically sophisticated age is the resurgence of good language and written skills, as we see happening on the Internet.

Doctor–patient relationships

In traditional face-to-face care there are two typical therapeutic relationship styles — the active–dependent relationship and the mutual participation, or partnership, relationship. With the evolution of online therapy, two new levels of relationship will evolve — the pre-therapy stage of self and family care, and the patient-driven relationship, where the doctor is merely an adviser, albeit an expert one. Armed with information, for the first time in history patients are able to "turn off" their doctor with the click of a mouse. This single factor will dramatically alter the power structure of the relationship.

In the traditional **active–dependent relationship** the physician is dominant, possibly even controlling and paternalistic, while the patient is mostly dependent and accepting. Patients have some choices, but they tend to play the role of passive follower behind an expert leader. This relationship is appropriate in certain online situations, especially early in the assessment process or when a clinician is using expert knowledge to advise on and teach about an illness. However, it will become less common in future as patients become increasingly empowered and knowledgeable.

The relationship of **mutual participation** is the ideal face-to-face relationship for most purposes. It implies equality, trust and collaboration, with both participants needing and depending on the other's input.

Now let's look at online relationships.

Online relationships

As patients become more knowledgeable, or "information rich", they will become the main driving force in the doctor–patient relationship.

E-health heralds a new **pre-therapy relationship** phase, where patients research, often with their family and friends, their problem or situation. Access to type 1 consultations will be particularly important here. It will become increasingly easy to discover high-quality reliable diagnostic and general information, but at the same time doctors will also be researched, as described in Chapter 6. All doctors of the future will have Internet homepages and patients will be able to make rational, informed decisions about the sort of doctor, and the type of relationship and treatment, that they want. In most cases patients will have carried out the research even before they have consulted the doctor, either face-to-face or online. Patients will be able to define when, how and where the relationship will occur and with whom. Doctors will have to lay out their wares, their skills, their products, to an increasingly savvy group of patients. Surgeons will detail their infection rates, physicians their drug interaction rates, and paediatricians their philosophies for treating children with cancer.

A physician colleague of mine who is an international expert on a very unusual disorder recently told me of his embarrassment when a company executive came to see him about his wife who was said to suffer from this particular disorder. He gave the executive the relevant information about the disease, quoted some papers he had written and explained how the man could best help his wife. To his surprise, at the end of the interview the executive suddenly produced a comprehensive list of 23 case reports of the disease taken from international literature on the Internet. The executive knew more about the recent case reports than did my colleague! Determined not to be caught on the hop like that again, my friend promptly installed an Internet connection in his office.

Of course many people will diagnose themselves before even seeing a therapist. There are a large number of good screening questionnaires on the Internet (check out the sites in the appendix). The beauty of these questionnaires is that you don't need a health professional to be present when you fill them in. Print out your results and discuss them with your doctor, as no such diagnostic tests are definitive. By filling out these questionnaires you may well facilitate your treatment, because your doctor will need to spend less time diagnosing you, leaving more opportunity for actual treatment and education about the condition.

In the fourth type of relationship the doctor is the adviser, while the **patient drives** the process of the relationship, makes the choices and the decisions, tapping into the doctor's expertise to create an overall treatment plan. The following example comes from my casebook.

I first met John, a 53-year-old married plumber, when he was brought into hospital by a squad of police following a siege. John was extremely paranoid and had started shooting at neighbours who he thought were being sent by the devil to kill him. Our initial relationship was an active–dependent one. On my orders John was sedated and placed in seclusion and was given medication. Over the next few days his psychosis settled but he became overtly depressed and felt extremely guilty about what he had done. As his paranoia decreased, our relationship started to become more equal. After leaving hospital he gradually gained in confidence, his mood improved with appropriate therapy and he and his traumatised family began to understand more about his illness.

I had diagnosed John as having a bipolar disorder — manic depression as it used to be known. He became an active member of a consumer support group, collaborating in his treatment and making his own choices as our relationship became one of mutual participation.

A year later John moved with his family to a town several hundred kilometres away. Although John now receives treatment and monitoring through a primary care physician, I still get occasional emails from him. These usually include the latest research findings in bipolar disorder with a request for my comments. For me this move to an online collaborator–commentator relationship is the evolution of a fascinating relationship. John now controls our relationship — quite the opposite of when we first met — and he makes sure I keep up-to-date with the literature on bipolar disorders!

The patient-driven phase of a therapeutic relationship is likely to become increasingly common as patients maintain long-term online relationships with their doctors. Patients who are interested in their own illnesses and keep up-to-date with the latest research and clinical findings through libraries and the Internet will feed information to their doctors, not only to keep the therapists up-to-date but, more importantly, to obtain the therapists' opinion of the new findings. And some of these relationships will be prolonged for years because of the ability of both patient and doctor to remain in contact via the Internet even after one of them has moved home, perhaps to a different country.

Communicating through our senses

One of the greatest human attributes is our ability to communicate — often with style and subtlety. We express ourselves with voice, language, gestures, face and body language, clothes and makeup, perfumes and hairstyles. We communicate to let others know about ourselves, to attract others and to make statements about how we see ourselves. Communication is the hub of all our relationships. In face-to-face situations we can see, feel, hear, taste and smell people. Despite a lack of scientific evidence, some people believe there is also a "sixth sense" — intuition, more commonly attributed to females than males.

In online relationships several of these senses are altered and we have to either do without them or depend more heavily on the other senses. This doesn't have to be a disadvantage. Blind people, for instance, compensate for their loss of vision by increasing their hearing and smell sensitivity and can often pick up environmental or relationship cues from those senses more accurately than sighted people. While the blind cannot see, they can still communicate effectively, albeit in a different way. This is what happens online.

We use different senses for the various different approaches to e-health. For example, on the telephone we use hearing only, often with a spicing of intuition thrown in. Many people feel less inhibited speaking on the phone and prefer it to communicating face-to-face. When we communicate using email or the Internet, we use our vision for the written word and other options such as videoclips, pictures and drawings. Hearing is important with Internet telephony and audible email attachments. Email is usually asynchronous communication with interactions occurring sequentially over hours or days, although chatgroups and netmeetings may be fully interactive.

Posted by Jerrie on bulletin board, September 1998

I have been with my partner for seven years and have always been faithful — until recently. A colleague at work began flirting with me on email. At first I took no notice but I was flattered and eventually I responded. I won't go into details, but once he gets what he wants he becomes very cold and accusing until, a few days later, the messages begin again. It's the detachedness of the situation, and the secret messages, that turns me on and keeps sending me back to him. I know he is using me, but what I don't understand is why do I repeatedly let him, and why do his messages drive me crazy for him.

Reply by Art

It seems to me that you are projecting all the qualities you look for in a partner onto your colleague. That is typical of online relationships because you cannot see or hear the other person, so the lack of stimuli and context makes your mind project the qualities you like onto others. Your colleague has proven to you that he is not what you thought he was. Do not jeopardise your solid relationship for a couple of weeks of excitement that will soon go. If you really care about your partner, end the online relationship — it's destined to fail sooner or later.

Communication online is obviously different from face-to-face communication. It will never be as comprehensive or integrated because it's unlikely we'll ever be able to smell or touch each other through a computer, although some researchers are now trying to "code" smells! But it does have some advantages. As our experience of the new technology increases, we will be able to communicate more effectively online. This will be a fascinating field for research.

Transference

The possibility of "transference" in online relationships should be recognised by both patients and doctors. Transference is the transfer of feelings from past events or relationships from the patient to the doctor. Counter-transference is the transfer of the doctors's feelings from past events or relationships to the patient. In the face-to-face world these feelings can be extremely powerful, to the extent that it is not uncommon for patients to fall in love with their doctors (or unfortunately, the reverse), or to act out extreme emotions such as anger, jealousy, rage and anxiety within the relationship. Sensible male doctors ensure that they have a female nurse with them during physical examinations if they are at all worried about this possibility. Falling in love with a patient is a major ethical sin for a doctor, and tends to lead to newspaper headlines, court cases and deregistration for the doctor.

In online relationships there is a higher likelihood of transference because the partners may not know as much about each other. This may be because the relationship is happening in only some sensory modalities or because the participants cannot pick up all the usual visual or other sensory cues. There is more uncertainty, more mystery, online. Patients project more readily onto their online doctor, as well as onto others with whom they are having online relationships. This leads to people reporting that everyone they meet online seems to be similar. They are not similar but are perceived as such because of similar projections onto them. Alternatively, the online user may be unconsciously picking up similarities in people that they meet online and self-selecting people for online relationships that fit with their own needs. These transference reactions are further complicated by transference to the computer itself, or to other communications technology which filters the doctor–patient relationship.

Transference and counter-transference are also seen in Internet therapy groups, as Yvette Colon describes (see "References and Further Reading"):

> *Unlike face-to-face group therapy, the online group exists only in time and mind. Because the group is available 24 hours per day and provides instant access to members who want to post when they are reflective or mad or inquisitive or thoughtful, response time is not always predictable. Because the group members and I did not see each other, it was easy for members to idealise me or project their fantasies and wishes onto me. Because I am unseen and "mysterious", anger and frustration were taken out on me more readily. Conversely my idealisation and projection onto clients could be difficult as well. Because I didn't know what the group members looked like, it became easy to accept the personas they created as the group continued.*

Our e-persona

We all have different personalities and, strange but true, our personalities can change when we are on the computer, especially when we are writing emails. As yet, we don't know much about just how different personality styles are affected by online technology or how different people react and behave in a variety of online situations. No doubt there will be plenty of research into this in the future.

What we can hazard a guess at, though, is how the different personality styles cited in the literature project themselves online. Take these, for example:

- **Psychopathic/antisocial personality**: Could these people be the online hackers and criminals — especially in deception and fraud — of the new millennium? Or are they the online "entrepreneurs" who pop up wherever there's money to be made and ethical principles are loose. Beware online "therapists" who might be in this category.

- **Narcissistic/self-loving personality**: Perhaps these people are running bulletin boards contributing at inordinate length as the "experts" and delighting in expelling everyone who disagrees with them. Maybe they're the ones who are heavily into cybersex — there's no chance of their losing face through premature ejaculation or rejection!
- **Avoidant/paranoid personality**: These people are probably lurking in the background of chatrooms watching everyone else or "flaming" (attacking) innocent email bystanders who they believe are threatening them.
- **Anxious/obsessional/dependent personality**: These people are probably meticulously organising webpages with accurate links and multiple layers of information. They are control freaks who spend a lot of time communicating with all and sundry in excessive detail so that recipients come to dread receiving their messages.
- **Histrionic/dramatic personality**: These characters have to be first in the newsgroup with the latest and greatest news. Unfortunately the news is often inaccurate or exaggerated. They're constantly demanding attention from online supporters, but only contributing when they can be the focus of the group. These people aren't likely to help anyone else online unless they can tell the world about it!
- **Dissociative/multiple personality**: These people are potential online disasters. If you can have multiple personalities in real life, the mind boggles at what could happen online. Perhaps they could run several groups all by themselves without the need for anyone else to contribute! This would be impossibly confusing for the average online doctor.

The important point here is that the online world allows patients and therapists an extension of their normal psychological world. Whatever their normal personality or coping styles are, these are likely to be exaggerated and magnified online. This is particularly so in text-only communication on the Internet where all sorts of identity fantasies can be acted out. It is common, for instance, for men to masquerade as women and to seek help for imaginary disorders from online doctors; and for both sexes to act out their sexual fantasies in the "safe" but very public Internet environment. Suler provides some fascinating examples of this in his excellent online book, *The Psychology of Cyberspace* (1996), at www1.rider.edu. In one example he describes how Brad met Natalie at a chatroom:

> *Brad was a college senior at an eastern university, she a junior on the west coast. They got to know each other better by corresponding through email. Over time, he felt very close to her. Maybe, he thought, he was even falling in love. When he finally suggested, then insisted, that he give her a phone call, the truth came crashing down on his head. Natalie confessed to being a 50-year-old man!*

Although this is superficially amusing, imagine how distressing it must have been for Brad. How it must have destroyed his confidence in himself. The increasing number of predators on the Internet is of great concern, and this is why e-doctors should know their patients' names. Anonymity on the Web in professional consultations is simply not appropriate.

The treatment process will change

There will be much more goal setting in e-health and treatment will be more goal directed than traditional treatment, and will focus more on information and education. In an ideal situation, the patient's goals will be carefully defined at the beginning of the consultation, and a treatment contract developed between the patient and the doctor to meet those goals over a period of time, ideally using a series of defined interventions and treatment guidelines. These will be connected to high-quality health information data bases which are easily accessible to the patient and individually tailored to their needs. The patients will be able to add to this database as they wish, because increasingly our health records will be stored in such a way that they are accessible to both patients and doctors via the Internet. Many of the multinational medical records companies are already producing electronic health-care records that can be accessed from the Internet, and Australia, for example, is at present considering the introduction of a national health information network which will allow all patients access to the majority of their health information. This will be another major driver of a changed doctor–patient relationship — of more empowered patients.

Patients are already regularly seeking other sources of help on the Internet apart from their usual face-to-face doctor. Dr Andy Lippman, the renowned futurist from the Massachusetts Institute of Technology Media Lab, notes how trusting people are on the Internet, commenting that people are quite prepared to take advice from unknown cyber-acquaintances. He uses the example of a friend of his who, needing urgent medical advice to help his child, went on the Internet, while his wife simultaneously phoned for the local doctor to come and see the child. On the Internet his friend discovered "Dr Flash Gordon" who said he was a doctor and emailed some simple advice to help the child. Dr Lippman said that his friend took this advice, which was accurate and helpful, and the initial crisis affecting the child was resolved even before the local doctor was able to get to his home. The back end of this story is that Dr Lippman later found out that he knew "Dr Flash Gordon". He happened to be a colleague living in the same building! It is fascinating how his friend had been prepared to trust an unknown person with the unlikely name of "Dr Flash Gordon" with the safety and health of his own child. There are many similar success stories of people who have used the Internet to seek help and assistance in what is essentially a global social support system. However, not all health professionals welcome these situations and some doctors positively fear the changes.

A little over a hundred years ago, many doctors reacted to the advent of the telephone with hostility. They worried that they'd be inundated with calls and that practising medicine over the telephone would somehow compromise their moral integrity and promote sub-standard care. In the same way, some doctors nowadays believe that practising health care over the Internet is inappropriate.

In fact, physicians were among the earliest users of the phone. The very first telephone exchange connected several Connecticut physicians to a central drug store and in the late nineteenth century telephone messages for doctors were often relayed through pharmacies. Alissa Speilberg (1998), from Harvard Medical School, draws parallels between the early days of the telephone and computer-based communications, particularly in terms of privacy and intrusiveness. She notes that "the telephone was particularly vexing to early users who complained of solicitations, eavesdroppers and even wire transmitted germs".

But by early this century doctors had learned how to screen calls and use intermediaries to assess call priority. And, Speilberg notes, patients and doctors learned how to use the phone more effectively, making patient–physician relationships "much more secure and private".

The beauty of email is that it has the potential to reach every physician, and in turn to be transmitted to all the physician's contacts, with quite ridiculous ease. Despite this, doctors and other health-care professionals have been relatively reluctant to use electronic communication in their practices, although this is changing rapidly. The reasons for this reluctance include the dread of being barraged by email and an even greater concern with privacy and confidentiality.

Interestingly doctors like myself who use email regularly do not find themselves snowed under by a deluge of messages. I find it easier to respond to patients' messages at my own convenience, and often with more consideration and care, than if I was answering a telephone call on the run. I now receive far fewer phone calls because patients and clinicians I work with know that they will get a reliable reply within 24 hours by email. This is much more efficient than the past games of "telephone tag".

Reviewing the ethical considerations, Alissa Spielberg (1998) concludes that "email use suggests a profound new social dynamic within the patient/physician relationship". She adds that email messages

> have the potential to be highly specific, descriptive and sometimes intimate portrayals of patient narrative and physician compassion … email communications are not merely virtual approximations of medical practice, they are very real exchanges of information, advice and emotions … The emergence of electronic communication launches a re-examination of the necessary values for good communication in the patient/physician relationship.

If accessibility, availability and a willingness to listen are the basis of good communication between patient and physician, then email facilitates all three bases. Email is quick and allows patients to go into as much detail about their concerns as they wish. Those patients who are intimidated by their doctor's office or reluctant or embarrassed to detail their feelings face-to-face often find it much easier to be honest using the written word.

Consumer needs

A number of researchers are starting to look more objectively at what are the real information needs of patients and carers, and what they want to find when they surf the Internet looking for health information. And it's not what you might expect. What is valued is interactive personalised information — not necessarily the most sophisticated or most scientifically presented. People want information that relates to them and their needs, and they want it delivered in as an immediate manner as possible, ideally through their doctor or another knowledgeable person. The health information that consumers want can be summarised as follows:

- answers to their specific questions
- results of their searches
- best sites for the topic
- disease "guides" (see below)
- consumer guidelines and FAQs (frequently asked questions)
- the ability to exchange email with their doctor or other knowledgeable people.

Equally importantly, there are certain types of information that are generally not valued:

- poor-quality, unreliable or biased information
- "shovelware" — traditional generic health information delivered pamphlet-style that is not interactive or personalised, and tends to be over-technical
- information that ignores the reality that most searches are performed by carers, not patients.

Consumer guides

Increasingly, good consumer-focused websites are employing "consumer guides" or "consumer mates". Two of the best-known sites taking this approach are http://www.canceronline.org and http://www.about.com. Consumer guides are patients who have had the illness that is the focus of the website and who work in partnership with the website itself, using their personal knowledge of the illness, and their extensive knowledge of the website, to literally guide other patients to information that is appropriate for them. Such guides may provide biographies of themselves. At Canceronline.org, for example, you email them direct, tell them a bit about yourself and your health problem, and they then email back and forth with you, suggesting information on the site, and possibly on other sites, that is appropriate for you. The guides are all accredited by the site and appear to be motivated by their wish to help others survive the illness that they themselves have had. Canceronline.org is a site of extremely high quality and is produced by a combination of physicians and consumers. This concept of consumer guides taking people around high-quality, reliable websites appears to me to be unbeatable. Let's hope we see much more of it in the future.

Digging up information for your doctor

Doctors can be quite threatened by patients who have discovered a large amount of information about their health, particularly from Internet sources. Some respond with confusion or bluster or in a dismissive or paternalistic manner; these doctors are usually ignorant of Internet health resources or assume that such sources are inaccurate. Others respond competitively. They take your information and rush off to the Internet themselves to prove that they can find more sources than you can.

Or they simply refuse to acknowledge that Internet material is valid.

However, many doctors are interested in what you have found, acknowledging that you might have more time to chase up unusual sources of information than they have.

So how do you approach your doctor if you have found what looks like useful information on the Internet?

First, tell your doctor that you are Internet literate and that you intend to search for information about your problem, or that you have already made such searches. Acknowledge that there is both good and bad information on the Internet and ask your doctor to help you judge the quality and reliability of the information that you have found. Explain the search strategy you intend to use, perhaps as indicated in Chapter 5, and you might find that your doctor is willing to learn that from you, as few doctors are trained to search sytematically. Make it plain that you will write a summary of the information that you have obtained and email this to your doctor before your visit. (No one wants to be presented with hundreds of pages of downloaded information which they are unlikely to find time to read.) Also ask whether your doctor knows any particularly good websites or other sources for your searches.

Searching the Internet and other online resources for valuable health information can be very time consuming, and a collaborative effort with your doctor is the best way to go. By following the above guidelines you are acknowledging that there is a vast amount of information available, that your doctor can't possibly know everything that is of relevance to your situation, and that you and your family are capable of becoming research assistants and librarians to help your cause. Your research can then be used by you and your doctor to develop a plan to manage your illness.

The following is an example of an email interaction between me and the parent of one of my patients.

Dear Peter — I found out about the possible use of fish oil for Miranda from www.schizophrenia.com. *There is another interesting site discussing Omega-3 fatty acids which seem to be the helpful element in the oil at* http://www.nimh.gov. *Can you follow up and see what you think so that we can discuss it when you next see Miranda? Thanks, John.*

My reply.
Thanks John — I have emailed the psychiatrist who is doing most of the research on fish oil and described Miranda's situation to him. Attached is a copy of our correspondence. He felt it would be worth giving Miranda a go on fish oil, given her continuing symptoms and only partial response to other medications. As you know, there are no guarantees, but it seems worth trying. You can buy it at most chemists as long as you tell them the seemingly active ingredient. I will find out something about dosing. Best wishes, Peter.

Peter — Thanks for your answer. I have discussed this with Miranda. You will need to ask her to take the fish oil as well — you know how much a typical teenager trusts her parents on things like medication! Will see you next week. Regards, John.

Blowing the cover on techno-speak

Doctors are famous for their technical jargon (and indecipherable writing, which online technology now eliminates). Two good examples of medical techno-speak are "dysdiadochokinesis" — to flip the hand backwards and forwards quickly — and "iatrogenesis" — the artificial causing of a disorder by health intervention!

Acronyms make the situation worse. In a medical record the notation "NBI" can mean either "No Bone Injury" or "No

Bloody Idea", while NAD can be "No Abnormality Detected" or "Not Actually Done"!

Now add the dreadful jargon of the information and computing environment. Terms such as "RAM (random access memory)", "legacy systems" (out-of-date systems that we can't afford to replace), "interconnectivity" (we'd love them to link, they should, but unfortunately they don't always), "closed systems" (can only be accessed by skilled hackers) and "best of breed" (the latest, greatest, and probably most expensive). And this is just a sample. Actually, a lot people who use these terms don't understand them themselves but fear they will appear stupid if they ask their meanings. I felt that way when I first got involved in information technology some years ago. Today, though, if there's a term I don't understand, I ask. This way, if the person using the term knows what it means, I get an explanation (and several thankful nods from people around me!), and if they don't, I treat everything they say with some caution.

You should always be able to understand what your online doctor is talking about. If you don't, ask!

A note on "netiquette"

Network etiquette, or Netiquette, is simply the customs and practices that guide the behaviour of Internet users. It is the online equivalent of good social behaviour, the ability to smile at people, shake their hand and look them in the eye when you talk to them. Unfortunately, many people do not practise good Internetiquette, perhaps because of the anonymity, yet immediacy, of the Web, but also through thoughtlessness. So what are the basic rules of Internetiquette?

1. First, apply the same standards you follow in real life to your behaviour online.
2. Familiarise yourself with any particular policies or procedures that

might be defined by websites you are searching, or individuals you are emailing. Some sites, for instance, specifically ask you to register, and to work through a series of processes, to obtain what you wish. What's wrong with going along with their request? This is particularly important when it comes to contacting individuals by email. As an example of this, I regularly get asked to review academic papers, or to be interviewed by students or journalists on email. I much prefer a polite note initially asking me if this is possible, and laying out broadly what will be expected of me, and I am generally quite receptive to such requests. A significant group of individuals, however, simply send me huge attachments to read and comment on, or, even worse, multiple questions that they want me to answer, without even asking if this might be convenient or possible. When they follow-up each week for several weeks afterwards demanding to know why I haven't done it, if I haven't, my blood pressure rises rapidly.

3. Think of other people's time, and of the bandwidth you are using. We simply cannot continue to use email in an exponential manner where the tendency is for people to send large attachments around to many folk just because it's easy. Equally, emails with fancy multimedia logos or signatures take up large amounts of room on computers. I regularly have to clean up the memory on my computer to eliminate the irrelevant files that have been received on email.
4. Be polite. If you get flamed, the chances are that you have broken the rules of netiquette. Unfortunately, "flamewars" can break out when many people start sending flames to each other. These are not only very upsetting but clearly also congest the network.
5. Try to avoid "SHOUTING". The convention of the Internet is that capital letters are used to show angry feelings. Apart from the fact that letters in upper case are often more difficult to read, you need to be aware of this convention.
6. If you are writing to somebody, do them the courtesy of including a descriptive header in your message. Once you start getting 60, 70

or 80 emails a day, as happens to me, you become very intolerant of people who don't tell you why they are contacting you.

7. Respect other people's privacy. Privacy is as important in the online world as it is in the real world. So only contact people if you think it is necessary. Contact that includes abuse in any form, particularly poor language or racist and sexist remarks, the sending of chain letters, broadcasting messages to massive lists, or actions that interfere with the work of other people are breaches of netiquette.

Emoticons

It is still difficult to fully show one's emotions when using email to interact. It is, however, possible to use a series of what are called "emoticons" that have emerged over the last few years by convention, on the Web, to identify your emotional state to your receiver. The following are examples:

: —)	User is happy	: — x	User's lips are sealed
: — (	User is sad	# —)	User partied all night
: — t	User is cross	: — 0	User is shocked

The email relationship

Deciding whether to have long-term or ongoing consultations by email is a major decision. Often you will write in great depth and length, with passion, confusion, anger or joy. It is somewhat like writing a diary except that the diary can write back. Most problems are quite complex and are not likely to be resolved overnight. It will take some time for you and your doctor or therapist to trust each other and to develop a therapeutic alliance or relationship. You need to be prepared to enter into a process of change and be honest with yourself and your therapist. All of this is much easier if your online doctor is also your face-to-face doctor, and your email consultations are of the type 2 variety.

There are three criteria for a successful email relationship: you feel comfortable using email and the Internet, you have the time for, and enjoy, writing, and you can write honestly and expressively about your feelings and reactions.

Dr Ellen Rothchild (1997), Chairperson of the American Psychiatric Association Telemedical Committee, comments on patient–doctor communication by email.

> [It] *holds promises and pitfalls. Email can be edited, printed and filed. Time zones and hearing and speech impediments become irrelevant. One message can go to many recipients. An emotionally needy patient with low tolerance for frustration in between appointments may be encouraged to commit thoughts to the word processor and email them between visits as an alternative to frequent phoning. Email, like web-surfing, can be exciting in its novelty and potential.*

John Suler, in his online book *Psychology of Cyberspace* (1996), looks at several other important issues relating to the way we communicate online:

> *When we are on the Internet we all tend to regress and act in a more child like manner. We tend to be less inhibited and more likely to act in primitive ways, in particular by "flaming" — attacking others who are online.*

The first online list I ever joined, for instance, which had been set up for health professionals only, demonstrated this perfectly. A person with differing political views from others on the list was flamed unmercifully and cruelly. By the time the list moderator tried to intervene, it was too late. Some very hurtful things had been said which would certainly not have been said face-to-face. The result was that many people, including myself, resigned from the list.

Sexual harassment is also unfortunately very common on the Internet. This is why you should be quite sure your online friends are who they say they are before you reveal any personal details. Despite all this, I am continually amazed at the lengths people go to help each other and by the remarkable generosity and warmth shown by so many to complete strangers, especially in chat rooms and on discussion lists.

The anonymity and asynchronous interaction of the Internet may cause problems. Because we can't see the person sending the message, and because they can use pseudonyms and addresses at Internet Service Providers, it is very difficult to identify individuals who want to remain anonymous. This anonymity amplifies the disinhibiting effect of email and can be good or bad depending on whether people are excessively rude or warm.

Email conversations don't usually occur in real time. They can take place over hours, weeks or even months. The advantage of this is that therapists and patients have more time to consider and evaluate their responses than in other therapeutic situations. When I receive emails that annoy me, unless they are very urgent I deliberately wait a day or so before answering. A considered reply is generally more valuable than an immediate one. Email communication means that plans and goals can be carefully designed, considered and reconsidered to achieve the best therapeutic outcome instead of everything being squeezed into a single, often rushed, consultation.

Using email, people can receive health education individually or in groups through open or closed chatrooms, secure or public spaces or lists, bulletin boards or support groups. One clinical educator can interact with many patient "students". Group work and information dissemination will also be greatly enhanced when easily downloadable videos using "videostreaming" techniques and videomail are introduced. It won't take the big health corporations long to work out the potential cost savings of providing online multi-party health education — estimated to take as much as 20 per cent of expensive conventional medical outpatient time.

Patients embracing change

There is no doubt that online technology will mean radical changes for both doctors and patients. But what do patients think about this? I've found that patients are not concerned about being interviewed or treated online. Patients often feel that e-health is more private than, say, a hospital ward where they may be asked intimate details of their personal and sexual life with only a curtain between them and several other patients.

In further evidence of patient acceptance Dr Warner Slack (1997) describes how over a five and a half year period 2,500 employees took part in computer interviews on their lifestyles at the Beth Israel hospital in Boston. The survey results included the following: 57 per cent of the employees reported high levels of stress, 43 per cent reported feeling "sad, discouraged or hopeless" in the previous month, and 6 per cent indicated that "life sometimes did not feel worth living". Of the participants 85 per cent responded positively to the computer interview, and when asked to compare the computer-based interview with an interview with a doctor or nurse, most participants preferred the computer.

In further studies Dr Slack discovered that patients being treated for alcoholism also found it easier to report high levels of alcohol consumption to a computer than to a psychiatrist; others were more likely to reveal sexual problems, a criminal record, impotence, being fired from a job or even suicide attempts to a computer than to a person. And more recently, in a 1998 editorial in the prestigious *Journal of the American Medical Association*, Dr Tom Ferguson noted:

Physicians may find it far easier than they think to offer their patients their own personalised blend of highly accessible, high quality, online health resources. In addition to welcoming patient email under appropriate circumstances, physicians might establish their own Web pages with lists of frequently asked patient questions and answers and annotated links to useful and authoritative medical Websites. Physicians could also provide biographical information, explain their practice philosophy, offer online appointment scheduling, and point to high quality health data bases and directories of online support groups. Such resources could serve current patients, help attract new ones, and might even allow physicians to budget their own time more effectively. Clinicians who invite their patients to join them in electronic conversation may reap another benefit as well — a better appreciation for the "other" side of their patient/physician relationship, which has commanded increased attention and has come under increased pressure in recent years.

The final word on email relationships should go to Gary Stofle, a social worker who has been providing email psychotherapy since 1996 on www.aol.com/stofle/onlinepsych.htm.

We can provide psychotherapy online. Human beings are wonderfully adaptable. We have found many wonderful and unusual ways of communicating with one another. For centuries we have used the written word to express thoughts, feelings and opinions with one another. We have used the written word to titillate, to persuade, to con, manipulate and harm others. And we have also used the written word to heal. Online psychotherapy is a way ethical therapists can use the written word to heal through establishing a therapeutic relationship.

CHAPTER 8

TELEPHOBIA, TELE-ADDICTION AND CYBERCHONDRIA

Nothing in life is free of risks and the Internet is no exception — especially where health is concerned. Most of the time the risks are just to do with poor information or advice, and the tips in this book will help with this problem. Even dishonest relationships can usually be indentified, although sometimes too late to prevent damage.

The potential risks for patients on the web can be summarised as follows:

- Internet addiction — excessive dependence on the virtual world
- poor advice, especially from anonymous chat rooms
- poor-quality information
- financial loss — through payment to poorly trained therapists, or for unproven therapies or health products
- dishonest relationships, where one partner in a relationship is deceitful about who they are, what they do, or what they wish.

However, there are some specific syndromes that are recognised by doctors and Internet researchers which merit special attention. Despite our move to cyberspace, many people are still scared of technology. That's telephobia. On the other hand, some people can't get enough of it. That's tele-addiction. And some people just go overboard in their worry about symptoms they have read about on the Internet. That's cyberchondria!

Telephobia

Despite living in the "information age", it is a recognised fact that more than half the population are frightened by technology. Can you program your video? Sure, we can all turn them on and off and do simple recordings, but anything more demanding is another story. And consider mobile phones and even the touch phones at home. How many people do you know who use all or even most of the options they offer? Is it that we are too lazy, not interested, too busy, or too afraid to work them out? And if we're baffled by mobile phones and video recorders, it is not surprising that computers and other hi-tech equipment are disconcerting.

Really, we only need to know as much about the technology as is required to accomplish our tasks. Of course, if we decide it's more interesting than we thought, we can always go further, learn more tricks and techniques, use more software. But for most of us it's just a matter of learning the basics of what we need. Forget about trying to work out what makes the computer tick. When we buy cars and lawnmowers we don't make their service manuals bedside reading. For some reason, many people think computers are different.

We all respond differently to new technologies, but for a considerable number of people they bring on a feeling of "technostress". According to Californian psychologists Dr Michelle Weil PhD and Dr Larry Rosen PhD (1997), technostress is:

> *the irritation we feel as our boundaries are constantly invaded by beeps, pagers and cell phone conversations ... It is our feeling that we should be able to work as fast as our computers. It is our bewilderment that with so many time-saving devices, we never have enough time. Technostress is our feeling of helplessness when our children or neighbours can 'surf the web' and we still do not know what that means!*

These sorts of stresses can lead to technophobias and telephobias. In his book *Technophobia* (1998), Mark Brosnan describes technophobia as "a resistance to talking about computers or even thinking about computers, fear or anxiety towards computers, hostile or aggressive thoughts about computers".

Some people with telephobia react to their often unconscious fear of the technology by shooting the messenger. They complain that the computer won't do what it's supposed to do, that the equipment isn't good enough and, in the case of many clinicians, that the patients won't like it. Many doctors also fear the changes to their practices that online technology will bring.

Fear of being online is usually associated with computers, but not exclusively. If you are the victim of a stalker, are receiving crank phone calls or expecting bad news, you may dread the telephone ringing. You may even refuse to answer it. I have seen patients in these situations who have become completely phobic about phones. One woman I knew eventually decided to do away with her telephone altogether. She associated phones with such dreadful news and distress that even having one in her home and office made her anxious. It made her job as an architect more difficult, but she solved the problem by using a messenger service to deliver handwritten letters between her clients and friends and herself. Luckily, her friends were very understanding.

Mark Brosnan (1998) suggests that technophobia is a legitimate response to technology and that this fear of technology is caused by social and cultural factors inherent in our society. Maybe it is a sense of social shame at their computer illiteracy that has led to thousands of American senior managers attending very expensive short courses in basic computing, often at secret exotic locations.

It has also been suggested that telephobia is related to old age. However, 14 per cent of people over 60 now use the Internet or email regularly, and there is little evidence that the elderly suffer more from telephobia. This is particularly important, as elderly people will benefit enormously from online home care.

We either love it or hate it!

People tend to fall into three distinct groups in their reaction to technology. Rosen and Weil describe us as "eager adopters", "hesitant 'prove its' " and "resisters". Which are you?

Eager adopters

Eager adopters love the technology. They view online activities as challenging and fun. I am one of these. Typically, I don't expect the technology to always be perfect, or even work, and I don't blame myself when it doesn't. The "eager adopters" include "nerds", computer salesmen and technology enthusiasts. Although this group makes up only 10 per cent of the population, most marketing is directed at it.

Hesitant "prove its"

Most people fall into this group, probably some 60–70 per cent of the population. They don't see online activities as much fun and only get involved when it can be clearly demonstrated that the activities are worthwhile. They're not into experimenting or sorting out their own online difficulties, preferring to call in help. This group will get a lot of use out of e-health, as long they concentrate on what they need and don't get bogged down with the technical side. People in this group are potential telephobics if they have bad experiences or don't receive the training they need. But their telephobias are eminently treatable. Most women fall into this category.

Resisters

Comprising about 20 per cent of the population, this group avoids technology as much as possible. Technology intimidates them. They tend to blame themselves when problems arise and this increases their feelings of inadequacy and fuels their determination to avoid online technology in the future. To cover their underlying anxiety, they tend to attack the technology. Some proudly call themselves "computer luddites" or "techno-luddites".

Am I telephobic?

How many of the following statements apply to you?

- I do not feel confident about operating a computer at a basic level.
- I am not interested in computer shops or product displays.
- I would not post an anonymous personal comment on an Internet bulletin board.
- I would not be prepared to email my usual doctor.
- I use the phone for necessary conversations only and do not like spending much time on it.
- I believe that information technology is greatly overrated in our society.
- Given the choice of a session on the Internet or a cold shower, I would choose the shower.
- I believe that the spread of information technology is a global attempt by big business to take over the world to satisfy their need to be in control.
- I do not like the idea of having a computer in my home.
- I will not enter a credit card number onto the Internet even if the site is meant to be secure.

If you agreed with four or more of the above, you may well be telephobic.

What can I do about it?

The best way to conquer a fear is to acknowledge that it exists, learn about it and then confront it. Some years ago I met a shark hunter and I asked him how he'd become involved in such an unusual occupation. His reply was that for years he'd been terrified of sharks and this was the only way to overcome the fear. Admittedly, his story is somewhat extreme.

There are two ways of overcoming telephobia. As a community, we need to change the way the technologies are presented so that they are more user-friendly and relevant. On a personal level, people may need to seek individualised help for specific problems.

Gender bias

Many more females than males are telephobic and it only takes a glance at the whole computer culture to see why. From an early age boys show more interest in computers — perhaps because computer store shelves are stacked with shooting, killing games which target males. In contrast there are very few games that appeal to girls.

Much of the advertising targets men. Most marketing is based on the computer's power. Is your RAM — random access memory — bigger and more powerful than mine? The parallel with the penis is exquisitely overt. What about the size of your "hard drive"? Is your modem fast enough to crash through the superhighway? Maybe the advertising gurus who dream up these slogans and macho advertising techniques don't realise that women may receive, often unconsciously, the reverse messages of rape and disempowerment. It is not surprising that so many women distrust technology.

Paradoxically, women actually use computers more than

men because of the predominance of women in secretarial roles.

Brosnan (1998) is in no doubt that the information industry's masculine bias is socially, not biologically, determined, which he says "can make computing motivationally problematic for feminine individuals (whether male or female)".

Women are not the only group in society under-represented in the computer industry; on a population basis black people are also under-represented, while Asians are significantly over-represented.

How changing the computer industry would help prevent telephobia

Feminising the industry and changing the culture

This is important. Until the masculine bias in the computer industry changes it will be hard to prevent many of the telephobic symptoms experienced by females. Girls as well as boys need to feel comfortable with computers from an early age. We need more computer software that interests girls. There needs to be a change in the attitude of teachers and in the content of courses in computing and information technology to make the subjects more appealing to females.

Changing the product and the marketing

The industry needs to identify a need and then design the product to fill it. At present the industry is infamous for its tendency to develop a new "toy" and then search out a market or a use for it — putting the cart before the horse. More market research needs to be carried out on how our lifestyles could be enhanced by the technology. Our needs should determine what products are created. The 90 per cent of people who are not "eager adopters" simply need computers that fulfill their basic requirements. Warner Slack (1997) sums up the situation perfectly. "When computer manufacturers ask 'How can we get physicians to use computers?' they are more likely to mean 'How can we get physicians to buy computers?' A better question would be 'How can we make our computers more helpful?' "

More collaboration and social conscience

The big players, such as Microsoft, Bell, Unisys, Macintosh and the like, need to develop a stronger social conscience, working together to use technological advances for social gain. (Less importance could be attached to market domination and obscene executive salaries.) When did you last see a multinational information technology company promoting social advantage as being as important as profits?

Socially responsible computer education programs

Currently computer education programs seem designed to produce propeller heads whose only desire is to write new programs or invent bizarre, incomprehensible acronyms. Of course this computer jargon is a great way of excluding non-members. We know very little about the effects of computers and particularly the Internet on society. What we need are education programs that concentrate on how the products affect society. Such programs are as important as the technological advances themselves.

Helping ourselves

It's unrealistic to believe that the computer culture will change overnight. We have to cope with our own fears and problems, and the following three broad approaches, used individually or together, generally work.

1. Give yourself time

You can't become comfortable with online technology overnight. As in any new situation it takes time to adapt and feel at ease. When we don't give ourselves enough time our natural defence is either to fight or flee. We end up getting angry with the technology, calling it "useless" or something much stronger, or running away. Both are effective short-term responses to our anxiety, but they don't do much for our long-term goal of learning to go online.

2. Obtain tuition using adult learning principles

We all learn best when given specific problems to solve in a supportive environment where non-judgmental help is readily available. For example, if you want to learn how to send email, the aim of the first teaching session should be to successfully send a simple email. Don't waste your time trying to understand what makes the computer work or the theory behind sending emails! Simply focus on how to accomplish the task. The extra "bells and whistles" can be covered in follow-up sessions. Countless people have been turned off using these technologies by being told to "sit down and get on with it — anyone can do it". Thankfully the boring software manuals of the past have been replaced with far more user-friendly onscreen "help" features.

3. Anxiety-reduction programs can help

These programs use desensitisation techniques to help phobic users relax when using a computer, or other technology, while at the same time allowing the individuals time to experiment safely online in a supportive situation. A fear response is replaced by a relaxation response. If you think an anxiety-reduction program could help you, look for Brosnan's book *Technophobia* (1998) which contains some sensible advice.

Alternatively, consult a therapist for a straightforward treatment program.

Tele-addiction

At the opposite end of the spectrum from the telephobics are the tele-addicts. The tele-addicts are the stuff of computer salesmen's dreams! Although "tele-addiction" doesn't yet appear in the American Psychiatric Association's Diagnostic and Statistical Manual of Psychiatric Disorders, there's no doubt it exists. It is also referred to as computer addiction, Internet addiction disorder, pathological computer use, technosis and cyberspace addiction. Rather paradoxically, an Internet support group for addicts, facilitated by John Suler PhD, has been set up at Psychology of Cyberspace at www.behaviour.net.

Most people in western societies will have read of cases of tele-addiction or know of people afflicted by it. There are always some people who will go overboard with any new experience. The online world provides a welcome escape for many people, but taken to the extreme it can affect normal social activity, family relationships and psychological development. Although most people believe that being online relieves loneliness, this may not be the case for everyone. A recent study from Carnegie Mellon University found that individuals who spent even a few hours each week online experienced greater levels of depression and loneliness than if they had spent less time on the computer! The researchers hypothesised that relationships maintained over long distances without face-to-face contact ultimately do not provide the kind of support that makes us feel secure and happy. Friends on the Internet aren't available to babysit at short notice, or have a cup of coffee. However, they felt that the Internet could be very successful in maintaining ties with friends who lived close by. Maybe we run into problems when we spend a lot of time keeping up relationships with people who live too far away for us to see much of. The evidence isn't in on this issue yet and more research programs are being undertaken.

There is substantial evidence that most computer addicts are males. Some researchers have gone so far as to suggest that it is only males who identify intimately with computers. This may seem far-fetched but, if true, the implications are mind boggling. Does this mean that males attach female characteristics to their computers and that the huge number of pornographic sites on the Web are proof of the computers sexuality? Or are socially avoidant males having relationships with asexual computer "mates" who have identical interests. It's probably safe to assume that if you have assigned your computer a name and personality you are showing signs of tele-addiction.

Advice columnists and other "agony aunts" receive many letters a week from women and men who are wondering whether to leave their spouse for someone they have met on the Internet. Many of these people will have isolated themselves in what Michelle Weil and Larry Rosen (1997) call their own "techno-cocoon", distancing themselves from the family unit. Of course, technology is not always the cause of the problem. The problem may be there already, and the Internet relationship just a symptom. Someone who feels isolated in the family unit may be drawn to the comfort of the Internet, further alienating themselves from their family and social system.

Internet activities are especially addictive. Surfing the Internet is rather like going fishing — one always expects to find the ultimate webpage in the next few minutes, just like one hopes to catch the largest fish in the river. When we do find a great website, possibly after hours of surfing frustration, our gambling instincts are reinforced and we carry on looking for the next "big win". Email users often have a tendency to check their mail several times a day. Evidence is now emerging that email may interfere with work and home efficiency, and enjoyment of life, if it is not carefully managed.

Virtual reality games, particularly those seen in arcades, are also addictive. They are carefully designed to appeal to the competitive element in people. Players have to continuously aim for higher levels of play, perform harder tricks, shoot more people or score more points. And while the games constantly reward success, very few people actually reach the highest levels.

On top of addictions, some of these games cause symptoms of the "post simulator syndrome". For instance, users of flight simulators sometimes experience illusions of turning or have difficulty walking after a prolonged "ride" on the simulator. These symptoms are so common that armed forces pilots are often actually restricted from flying real aeroplanes for between 12 and 24 hours after "flying" a simulator. Although virtual reality three-dimensional games, and clinical virtual treatment programs, are still fairly uncommon, it may well be that in the future when they are widely available there will be a requirement to restrict driving or operating heavy machinery for a few hours after being in a virtual environment.

How to recognise a tele-addict

Addictions are simply behaviours over which we have little control. They can cause us distress or disrupt our lives personally or socially. It is easy to see how this can happen in cyberspace. The desperate wife of an addict recently posted this note on the Internet:

> *I'm so angry with all of you out there. You've taken my husband from me. He won't talk to us anymore because he lives in a fantasy land — the same fantasy land that you're all in!!!! Snap out of it!*

Live your lives and speak to people face-to-face. He doesn't think there's a problem. He's on all night — he doesn't know his family anymore. I'm so desperate I'm calling on you to reply to me so I can show him what you think and hope that he wakes up to himself. He might believe something you say cos he won't believe me. I can't believe I am asking you people in cyberspace to help me get my husband back to the real world.

Recently Dr Kimberley Young PhD published a book entitled *Caught in the Net* (1998), in which she describes the following eight signs as being typical warnings of Internet addiction and suggests that five or more positive responses may indicate addiction.

- Do you feel preoccupied with the Internet (think about previous online activity or anticipate the next online session)?
- Do you feel the need to use the Internet for increasing amounts of time in order to achieve satisfaction?
- Have you repeatedly made unsuccessful efforts to control, cut back or stop Internet use?
- Do you feel restless, moody, depressed or irritable when attempting to cut down or stop Internet use?
- Do you stay online longer than you originally intended?
- Have you jeopardised or risked the loss of a significant relationship, job, educational or career opportunity because of the Internet?
- Have you lied to family members, therapist or others to conceal the extent of involvement with the Internet?
- Do you use the Internet as a way of escaping from problems or of relieving a dysphoric mood (feelings of helplessness, guilt, anxiety or depression)?

Not everyone takes Internet addiction as seriously as Young does. The following list of signs of Internet addiction are found at Netaholics Anonymous (www.safari.net).

You wake at 3 a.m. to go to the bathroom and stop and check your email on the way back to bed.

You get a tattoo which reads "This body best viewed with Netscape Navigator or higher".
You name your children Eudora and Dot.com.
You spend half of the plane trip with your laptop on your lap ... and your child in the overhead compartment.
Your hard drive crashes. You haven't logged in for two hours. You start to twitch. You pick up the phone and manually dial your Internet service provider's number. You try to hum to communicate with the modem. You succeed!!

"Online-aholics"

In her book Young describes the results of her survey of 396 "Internet addicts" and in particular notes the effect of the behaviour on their spouses, partners and families. She suggests that those most likely to become "online-aholics" are people who already suffer from anxiety, depression and low self-esteem or who have had previous addictions. Exploring the reasons why so many teenagers and students become Internet addicted, or nerdlike, she concludes that the combination of unstructured time, free Internet use and particular personality traits is a potential disaster. Young says that young people with socially avoidant, isolated or obsessional personality styles seem to be most at risk, with the online addictions often leading to plummeting grades and damaged social lives.

No-one knows how many people have tele-addictions or exactly what sort of people they are. In his online book *The Psychology of Cyberspace* (1996) Dr John Suler comments that "so far researchers have only been able to focus on trying to define the constellation of symptoms that constitutes an Internet addiction", never mind trying to properly research all the other facets of the disorder. He concludes that there is a problem "when your face-to-face life becomes dissociated from your cyberlife" and notes the important corollary that "It's healthy when your face-to-face life is integrated with your cyberlife".

Posted by Newbie, September 1998
Hi, I'm new here and I have a problem. I am sixteen years old and am involved in an online relationship with a girl who lives in Michigan. Almost every day we meet in a chatroom. Then one day she didn't turn up and I got worried. She didn't respond for two weeks. I went to some of the websites she visits and posted "missing persons post" in guestbooks and message boards. I and some of my friends emailed her for two weeks but still there was no reply. Eventually she replied to say that she had gone on vacation for 2 weeks and telling me to get a life and leave her alone. She told me she had found some new friends and wasn't going to hang out on the Internet so much in future. She said she thought I should do the same. This made me think because I was so upset. I just realised that I don't have a life because I spend so much time online — like 8–12 hours per day. My family is suffering from financial and money problems and I've been turned down for jobs. My parents won't let me drive the car (insurance problems) so I basically don't go outside the house and I had nothing better to do than go online. The pain of losing her is so bad — she wants me to leave her alone and I must respect her wishes. I feel like a tortured soul.This is tearing me up. Thanks for reading this and giving me some advice.

Reply by Anita
Hi — I can really relate to what you say. I have "dated" 4 guys off the Internet. I know it is really easy to think you have fallen in love with someone over the Internet, but trust me, it's not the same. I have even had supposed boyfriends send me pictures of them that weren't even them!! You are young. You may not like to hear this, but what she said is right. It's hard to have a normal relationship on the Internet. I am engaged to a guy I met on the Internet, but we agreed not to make any commitments until we met in person — that was smart and safe. And the good thing is that we both do lots

of other things away from the Internet although we both still really like it. I don't think your relationship would have gone too far, and even though you've had a bad experience if you take the advice it might turn out for the best in the long run. I hope I've helped ya just a little.

Cyberchondria

This is one of the most recent words spawned by the Internet, and it means a form of Internet addiction driven by anxiety. We all get somewhat hypochondriacal on occasions, and believe that we have illnesses where none exist. Patients with "hypochondria", having heard tales of woe from a friend, a colleague or the local gossip, believe that the minor symptom they have may be a sign of impending doom and a long and prolonged death. Medical students often worry that they have symptoms of the diseases that they study. A proportion of them regularly end up seeing dermatologists, worrying about their own spots and lesions, soon after they have studied skins, or get their eyes checked after an ophthalmology term.

It's quite natural that if we suddenly have access to huge amounts of health information, that we might start imagining that we have dreadful illnesses. There is no doubt that some patients are presenting with symptoms of "cyberchondria". "Treatment" generally consists of providing reassuring and accurate information about their health status, and teaching them how to work with their doctor and analyse the health information that they found on the Web more critically. I treated one young man, a very intelligent university student, who had to be literally withdrawn from the Internet because he was spending up to 18 hours a day searching for "cures" for his fantasy illnesses. Luckily he had understanding parents who did not have a computer at their home and who let him move back with them for several months so that he could be "dried out" in an Internet-free environment.

Preventing or treating the addiction

Information about the treatment and prevention of tele-addictions is thin on the ground, presumably because they have only recently been recognised. The only therapy centre I have found that specialises in treating tele-addictions is the Centre for On-Line Addiction which is run by Dr Young.

However, there are four principles that underlie the treatment of any addiction. These are:

1. Acknowledge and recognise that the addiction is a problem.
2. Control and/or cease the addictive activity or behaviour.
3. Replace the activity or behaviour with a more healthy alternative.
4. Assist other family members or friends who have been affected by the addiction.

Recognition

Most addicts use projection ("It's everyone else's fault") and denial ("I don't do it anyway — it's not a problem") as psychological defence mechanisms, whether their addiction is smoking, alcohol or sex. To get past this and to get a picture of the extent of their addiction the addict is asked to keep an objective diary of their Internet behaviour. Their partner (who is inevitably more angry and more truthful) may also be interviewed and asked to help in this process.

I have devised a simple questionnaire to detect tele-addiction based on one designed and used world-wide to identify alcohol addiction. You can slip these questions into normal conversation with someone you suspect is tele-addicted, to identify their level of addiction. I have named this the **RAGE** test for tele-addiction.

- Have you unsuccessfully tried to **R**educe your use of the Internet?
- Has anyone been **A**ngry with you because of the amount of time you use the Internet?
- Have you felt **G**uilty at the amount of time you use the Internet?
- Have you **E**scaped from social activity to use the Internet at inappropriate times?

This test requires further scientific validation, but, if one draws on the equivalent alcohol test results, people scoring 3 out of 4 would have about a 60–70 per cent chance of becoming tele-addicts at some stage in their lives. Those who score 4 out of 4 would have an 85–90 per cent chance. Try it yourself and see what you think!

Control or cessation

Most addictions are best treated by controlling the behaviour; only in exceptional circumstances, where considerable damage is being caused, must people stop the behaviour altogether. Tele-addicts should try to modify their behaviour by restricting their access voluntarily. If this doesn't work, pull out the power plug! Concentrate on other activities for a while then try again at a later stage to reintegrate online activities into your lifestyle.

One patient I recall only managed to reduce his Internet activity when he was made to pay a fine of $5 an hour to the charity of his choice once he went above an agreed one hour per day of online activity. He rapidly learned that he couldn't afford to keep up the activity. The importance of money as a motivator and driver of human behaviour should never be under-estimated.

Controlling the behaviour runs into problems when people "fall in love" with their computer. Dr John Suler (1996) calls the phenomenon a "transference reaction to computers". Transference, where the patient transfers patterns of thinking and feelings from past relationships to current relationships, is common in online relationships and is discussed in Chapter 7. But transference to a computer! It does happen. The incidence of people who give their computers a name and personality is extremely common! I hope this won't be your reaction to your computer failing:

> *Lisa's crashed again — she doesn't like wet weather — her hard drive just can't take it. I've got to get her repaired quickly so she can feel OK again. I feel so guilty if I don't look after her properly. It's typical that this should happen now just when I had her hooked up with a really good printer.*

Computers can be loved children, as in Lisa's case, powerful parents, erotic partners, good listeners, uncritical friends or can even become part of one's own identity. These computer relationships are often a substitute for unfulfilled needs; while not inherently harmful, they can become so if they become unrealistic, excessive or too intrusive. If people are receiving e-therapy from one of the many counsellors on the Internet, transference reactions to the therapist and to the computer may need to be explored and acknowledged as part of the therapeutic process.

Behaviour replacement

If you are attempting to reduce the time you spend online, it's important to find fulfilling activities to replace the online activity. The best approach is to look back at what you used to do before you discovered online activities, and what interests you lost as a consequence of your tele-addiction. Some people will want to take up these interests again, whereas others will move in different directions. Much online activity takes place late at night, and it is worth finding out why the computer is preferred to bed! Stories abound of people in unsatisfactory relationships using online activity as a substitute for these relationships. Others use the computer to develop relationships with new partners.

Esther Gwinnell, in her fascinating book *Online Seductions* (1998), gives many examples of people falling in love with strangers on the Internet, including the following letter from "Estherg" to "RainGoddess". Estherg is spending huge amounts of time on the Internet relationship. Attempting to get her to restrict her online activity would presumably be very difficult.

> *I have fallen in love with a man I met on the Internet — at least, I think it's love. Can it be real love? I've never met him, but we exchange 20 emails a day and spend hours on the phone. I've seen his photograph, and he really turns me on. Frankly my heart just skips a beat when I see his name in my email list. He seems to have everything I want in a man, and I think I love him. But it scares me — how can this be real love? Over the computer? Never having met? Do you think someone can fall in love like this?*

One can only imagine how much time it takes to exchange 20 emails per day.

Helping the addict's family

Anger. Jealousy. Envy. Exasperation. Fury. Suspicion. Resentment. Mistrust. Loss. Hopelessness. These are the sorts of emotions commonly reported by the partners or family of tele-addicts. Mostly what they want is the return of a loved one, but they also have many issues to work through, not least being the changes they will have to make to their own lives once the tele-addict abandons his or her addiction and has more time for others. How will they cope with this? How has their own life changed to cope with the tele-addiction and do they really want it to go back to how it used to be? If not, what changes do they need to make to ensure that the future is satisfying for themselves and their "recovered" partners?

Family members can find help through Internet support groups such as the Internet Addiction Support Group at www.behaviour.net, although the Internet might be the last place some of these people would look for help!

Unfortunately all the advice in the world may not be enough if either the computer or the online activity has become part of an individual's identity and reason for being. An anonymous college student put it this way during a chat group:

> *It's what I am. Everyone knows me as a computer nerd, and I'm proud of it. It's the only thing I've ever been really good at. I love my computer. Lots of people come to me for advice and it makes me feel really good to be able to help them. Why even the girls who used to ignore me now ask me to help them. It's really important for me to keep my website up to date — everyone thinks it's so cool.*

So be careful!

CHAPTER 9

"LEAD, FOLLOW OR GET OUT OF THE WAY" — WHAT DOES THE FUTURE HOLD?

The way most doctors and health-care professionals do their jobs has hardly changed over the past thirty to forty years. Contrast this with the enormous changes in, say, transport, manufacturing and telecommunications.

But hang on to your stethoscopes! Despite the fact that most doctors still have their heads buried firmly in the sand, the winds of change are blowing around them. Sooner rather than later they will be exposed. The combination of technological change, the demands of business and the rise of consumerism are causing radical changes in the way health care is practised around the world. E-health is poised to revolutionise health practices. The changes will be the 21st century's equivalent of the public health initiatives of sanitation and nutrition which revolutionised health care in the 20th century. The integration of online technologies will allow doctors and patients to work together on electronic health records, with patients having much more say in their treatments. The development of Internet 2 and videomail (video clips sent like email) will bring e-health into everyone's home. People will be treated in "virtual hospitals" by global clinicians. As Dr Rick Satava (1996), who has worked with the NASA medical space program for some years, said, "the future isn't what it used to be".

A recent study by Mercedes Benz shows that 12-year-olds using paddles, as are used in Nintendo games, drive cars better than adults using steering wheels. As a result, the day might not be far off when cars are produced with paddles for steering and the steering wheel is but an optional extra! The way we interact with communication systems is going to radically change the way we behave and think in ways that are impossible to predict. And the computer-literate children of today will drive these changes.

Nobody can say with any certainty where or how far the information revolution will take us — not even the computer and information experts. Five years ago they thought they knew, but huge advances in information technology have taken them by surprise. Unable to anticipate the changes, the experts are now finally asking the users what they want. This means that, in the health arena, patients and clinicians need to make their demands clear. We must say what we want.

It's a changing world

In the past, land, capital and people have been seen as the economic cornerstones of our society. To these add "knowledge". The storing of, and passing on, of knowledge from one generation to the next has impacted mightily on the development of the world. Consider the Bible; it was written two thousand years ago but is still the most widely read book in the world. Every day all over the globe its teachings continue to influence people.

Knowledge has never been as important — and as accessible — as it is today. Bruce Bond, charismatic recent chief executive officer of Picturetel (a multinational videoconferencing company), describes the present as a "wrinkle in time". He sees world-wide changes caused by the development of the information and communication industries as being a sort of dividing line between two periods of time. His thesis is that living on one side of what will probably be a 50-year "wrinkle" which started around 1980 will be completely different from living on the other side.

Bond describes the changes as "evolutionary, revolutionary and devolutionary".

The evolutionary processes within "the wrinkle" are the new tools — the hardware and software of the computer industries — and changed business processes.

The revolutionary changes relate to the easier access to information and knowledge, leading to fringe companies or activities replacing traditional centralised organisations. Already small Internet companies created by young, adventurous people are springing up overnight and challenging the multinationals. The equivalent in health care will be the really good online doctor who might live in, for instance, Montreal, Canada, but who, because of her globally recognised skills, knowledge, empathy and expertise, attracts patients from all over the world. Many of her patients would have previously gone to local teaching hospitals which will now have to compete on a much more level playing field.

The devolutionary changes predicted by Bond will see organisations becoming more localised and less hierarchical. It is only in the last 150 years that we have built hospitals that are monolithic, hierarchical institutions with complicated administrative processes. These hospitals are not only threatening to, but can be quite dangerous for, patients — evidenced by the number of patients who contract hospital-acquired infections or "iatrogenic" (doctor-caused) diseases. Over the next fifty or so years many large hospitals, as we know them, will disappear, leaving only a few centres of expertise staffed by super-specialist doctors and other health professionals. Thousands of people each year die as a result of medical mistakes in our hospitals, but this should be reduced once we have better information systems that are easily available to all of us. Health care will have become a distributed enterprise. We will be able to concentrate our scarce health resources on wellness promotion, instead of just the treatment of illness. There will be more resources available to undertake, for example, the mass immunisation campaigns that are needed around the world and which have in recent times been promoted by the Gates Foundation, a billion-dollar philanthropic organisation funded by Melinda and Bill Gates.

It's a shrinking world

Within the next few years it won't matter where we are in the world, we will be able to access e-health as described in this book. This is due to two technologies, fibre-optic cabling and satellites. Already 500,000 kilometres of fibre-optic cable connect cities and countries around the world. This will double within the next five years. By the end of the year 2000 the latest of many intercontinental data links, a massively powerful fibre-optic cable weaving from Germany through the Mediterranean, across Southeast Asia and on to Japan and Korea, will be installed. Most of this cabling is to accommodate the Internet. The slow part of the Internet is still the switches that direct data in different directions around the world, but these too are being speeded up using light and laser technologies, and the switches of the near future will be able to handle the equivalent of the entire volume of data carried by today's Internet in just a second or so!

At the same time, improved interactive satellites are being launched. Acting like mobile phone towers, or repeaters, they provide world-wide coverage. At present there are just over two hundred such satellites in "low earth" orbit, but within five years there should be more than a thousand. As the bandwidth or "pipes" broaden, real-time interactive video will be available all over the world. People will be able to talk and see their mum, their dad, their friends or their doctor on their home monitor anytime they want. And the monitor may be a TV or a computer, or on the fridge, the microwave, or perhaps hanging on the wall like a picture! And if you are out and about you will use your phone to see and speak to people using WAP technology (wireless application protocol).

The two "pipelines" complement each other. Fibre-optic cables enable information and data to pass very quickly from one point to another; satellites provide total coverage. The world is being quietly wrapped in a cocoon of communications that will support Internet 2 to bring health care ubiquitously to your home.

What is Internet 2?

We must build the second generation of the Internet so that our leading universities and national laboratories can communicate one thousand times faster than today. But we cannot stop there. As the Internet becomes our new home and town square, a computer in every home — a teacher of all subjects, a connection to all cultures — this will no longer be a dream but a necessity.

President Clinton in his 1997 State of the Union address

The Internet 2 consortium is made up of people from more than 130 mainly American universities and 44 commercial partners. It has three main goals:

- to enable a new generation of applications
- to recreate leading-edge research and educational network capability
- to transfer that capability to the global population.

The partners have each made significant financial commitments to Internet 2 and have agreed:

- to build their campuses or companies to connect internally and externally at at least 100 megabyte speeds which will allow almost any video or audio application
- to support their staff or faculties in learning how to work with Internet 2
- to share their findings with the commercial world.

As a consequence, Internet 2 will have major benefits. More and better quality information will be available in high-quality video and audio; virtual reality systems will create a dynamic rather than the current static environment; the wide band will facilitate better exchange of ideas, collaboration and communication in real time; and information delivery will be more reliable.

Internet 2 will radically change the way we work, play and do business. It is particularly exciting for health. We will be able to develop fully digitalised libraries which include not just text but comprehensive video and audio collections. We will build collaborative virtual research laboratories enabling "tele-immersion" — the ability to move inside space, inside the human body and into virtual reality situations, where several people can share space at the same time. Douglas Van Houweling, chief executive officer of the Internet 2 consortium, has already demonstrated how surgeons and students will be able to immerse themselves inside a three-dimensional virtual middle ear, allowing the surgeons to teach the anatomy, pathology and surgery of the ear to their students inside that organ.

The Internet 2 (http://www.Internet2.edu) will open up collaborative opportunities as yet undreamed of. Online health services will be developed for patients, as well as teaching, educational programs and research activities. We will learn more about medical disorders as world experts are able to communicate in virtual space and time much more easily. As a researcher in schizophrenia I will be able to access the latest research data as it is produced around the world. Research programs will become truly global as databases from around the world are combined to better understand the epidemiology of disease. Virtual laboratories and social environments will be constructed, giving us a much better understanding of the experience and effects of illness, and a more effective measurement of the various treatments.

Combine the communications revolution with the genetic discoveries associated with the largest international scientific research project in the history of the world, the Human Genome Project, where our genes are being explored and typed, and the prospects for future health care are amazing and exciting. The field of genomics, which uses our genetic knowledge to prevent and treat illness, will combine with the fields of nanotechnology and robotics, where minituarised physiological and other manufactured devices will be able to be programmed to literally operate on us from inside our bodies. And these exciting advances will be supported by the communications revolution that is just commencing.

E-healthcare for the new millennium

Institutions and paper medical records will be a thing of the past. The patient will come first. Wellness will be promoted, patients will receive continuous care in the community in an active partnership with their doctors. Computerised records owned by patients and shared with their doctors will tie everything together. Paperless hospitals, like those recently developed in Malaysia, will be common. In time the computer, television, telephone, telemedicine systems and other technologies will be integrated into a single interactive communications technology. No one has thought of a good name for this yet. Perhaps "the telefusion" would be a good one. This "telefusion" device will be linked to the Internet 2 and will be on every doctor's desk. Health-care professionals will use it to access patient records, to videoconference with colleagues and patients, to link to library, financial and administrative programs and systems and to attend to all their personal requirements too.

Not everyone will have a "telefusion" device at home, but, just as we have commercial 'Internet cafes' now, I believe public "telecentres" will spring up where people will be able to access their records or use other parts of the Internet. This will be especially important in the underdeveloped nations, where the communications revolution will allow much more rapid social and economic development than would otherwise have been possible.

Major teaching hospitals will not escape the winds of change. As Internet 2 effectively spreads knowledge to every corner of the globe, there'll be less need for teaching hospitals in every city. Instead, I suspect that teaching hospitals or tertiary field centres, servicing whole states or countries, will emerge to provide super-specialist procedures not available in community-based centres.

These tertiary centres will service not only countries but international time zones. Up until now we have got on pretty well by carving the earth up into continents and countries. However, the world of the future is more likely to be divided into three different time zones, because, despite all our accumulated knowledge, we still haven't found a way around the need for human beings to sleep! It is unlikely that clinicians in a major tertiary hospital in, for instance, New York will want to service patients in India who are in an almost opposite time zone. These three time zones are likely to comprise, first, North and South America, second, Europe, Western Russia, India and Africa, and third, Eastern Russia, Asia and Australasia.

It will be interesting to see if a major teaching hospital in Rio de Janeiro is able to compete with an equivalent institution in Washington, DC, to provide services to patients in Mexico!

Present-day health businesses are mostly a hotchpotch of small cottage industries, powerful autocratic empires, or protected, poorly defined heirarchies that not even the doctors who work within them can understand. Just as businesses have become more flexible, and major companies have become enterprises, partnering with each other in different ways at different points in time depending on their needs, so health-care groups will become enterprises. This added flexibility will provide more choice for patients as these health enterprises expand and contract in response to clinical demands and needs rather than through historical forces.

This approach will demand significant efficiencies, and changes, in the training and practice of all health professionals, especially doctors. Medical schools and other health-care education institutions will have to entirely change their teaching curricula. Being the Dean of a medical school, typically a conservative profession, will be very difficult over the next 20 years.

Although clinicians have embraced some communication technologies, such as telephones, mobiles, faxes, pagers, tape recorders and TVs, computers have not been put to good clinical use. Instead they are mostly used by doctors for accounting purposes. This is a reflection of the narrow reductionist government policies aimed at controlling costs and increasing profits rather than improving the quality of patient health care.

Shopping around

As the brave new world emerges there is no reason why you shouldn't "visit" a surgeon, nutritionist, physician or nurse based in different areas around your country or global time zone. Multidisciplinary health-care teams, preferably coordinated by your local primary-care face-to-face doctor are inevitable. This will mean, over time, a complete re-engineering of health systems both inside countries and globally. In the United States this will cause major difficulties because of the entrenched positions by all of those with a stake in the old system — the obscene profit-driven Health Maintenance Organisations (HMOs) and the lawyers who put up the cost of medicine dramatically by constantly facilitating legal suits against doctors, who defensively respond by over-ordering tests and investigations to protect themselves, at the patients' cost.

The arrival of Internet 2 will leave these health vultures high and dry in their well-feathered nests. Whether they like it or not, Internet 2 will put video e-health activities on everyone's desktop wherever they may be in the world. It will be fascinating to see how this affects the US health-care industry. Will we see true international competition in health? Physicians in Australia typically charge between US$60 and US$80 an hour, which is half that charged in the United States. Market forces are likely to dictate fee rates. Some patients will choose cheaper treatment by equally qualified overseas doctors. As a potential consumer, I have no problem with seeking an opinion from a world expert situated, say, in London, New York or Toronto. If they also happen to be cheaper than my local physician, I am doubly blessed.

Obviously, issues of policy, legality and medical registration will need to be sorted out around the world, as most doctors and other health professionals are registered only within their own countries. But this will happen. Consumers will demand that it happens.

Patient power

We are living not only in the age of information technology but also the age of consumerism. For many reasons, the area of health has not been greatly affected by the rise of consumerism — but this is about to change. Patients must become more involved in the debate on the future of e-health and health-care delivery. They are the pivotal points in a system that has, for so long, focused mainly on the needs of clinicians. Curtis Rooney, a health-care lawyer from Washington, proposes a "patient's bill of rights". "Nothing should limit the ability of an individual to obtain advice from any health professional licensed within the United States." This is a great idea except that it should take on a global perspective. Why shouldn't an online patient in Russia have the same rights as one in Baltimore?

Dr Tom Ferguson, one of the medical gurus of the consumer movement, has long been critical of the type of health information provided by doctors to patients, calling it "shovelware". Shovelware consists of the typical patient information pamphlets that you see in your doctor's office, often produced by drug companies, and offering generic, and very general, information. Ferguson has researched the type of information patients want, working with a very, in his words, "net-savvy" group of health consumers. The results are commonsense. Patients want replies to their specific questions, individualised information presented interactively, the results of health searches that are specific to their problem and information about the best sites for their problem. Increasingly consumers also want to access a “disease mate” or “consumer mentor” who has the same problem, and who can lead them to the relevant health information in a sensitive manner (see Chapter 7). The emergence of better health information and consumer mentors will change the way patients understand their diseases and will greatly assist the majority of patients in their quest for good treatment. What examples of patient power!

The wider benefits for all of us

The tangible benefits of e-health are already obvious. The Baby Care Link telemedicine program managed by Dr Charles Safran at the Beth Israel Hospital in Boston is a good example. Premature babies in intensive care are linked by videoconferencing to their parents at home. The parents can phone up any time of day or night to see and interact with their children. In this case telemedicine is being used to provide emotional, educational and medical support to families of hospitalised babies. It will also facilitate bonding and reduce the potentially damaging long-term psychological effects of prematurity and parental separation over the first few months of life. This sort of facility will soon be available to all of us as bandwidth increases and we can access video on the Internet.

In the future, families will be able to make video visits to loved ones in hospital when it is not convenient to visit, saving time and energy. And video visits will not only be confined to hospitals; whenever we are away from home on work, holiday or even in prison, we will be able to keep in touch by video. The videophone, or telefusion instrument, is going to change our lives more than we can possibly imagine as we discover more and more applications for it. It really will be a case of “seeing is believing”.

Teaching our children well

Children, more than any other group, have embraced online technology with a passion and we shouldn't pass up this golden opportunity to instill healthy lifestyle habits. By the time they turn twelve most children have already acquired lifelong behaviours. After this, many "switch off" learning new life skills of a preventive nature. Fortunately their brains "switch on" again when they reach about twenty-five, but by that time a proportion will have already suffered many life traumas — such as drug and alcohol abuse, relationship break-ups and instability, or unwanted pregnancies. Yet this is a time in their lives that should be exciting and fun.

Children in western countries are quite at home on computers. Unfortunately most computer games are "mindless" and teach them little more than how to manipulate a joystick or keyboard. What we must do is develop challenging and exciting computer games and online programs which deliver effective health-care and lifestyle messages. We know that even very young children are highly receptive to educational messages. Marketing is crucial and can be seen in the success of companies such as McDonalds and Coca-Cola who, through aggressive education and marketing campaigns, have managed to become part of our children's culture, causing lifelong behavioural and psychological dependence on, and interest in, "junk food".

We need to move beyond the "quit smoking" campaigns to online education campaigns which prevent people from taking up smoking in the first place. This is one of the primary aims of the Centre for Online Health at the University of Queensland. Over the next few years the Centre will be developing "child friendly" educational multi-media games for primary school children that will be fun to play but which will also carry preventive health messages. These programs will be used as part of the school health curriculum, facilitated by teachers, and will involve families and communities, not just children, as health interventions as well as health education. Perhaps one title might be "Doom defies Dope"! A great title to use to explore the importance of power in relationships and to teach children and families about ways of avoiding abuse and violence. The use of online technologies to improve the health prospects of the next generation is an exciting prospect and within our grasp.

A better understanding of illness

If doctors were able to feel at first hand what their patients were going through, the benefits would be enormous. The first time I experienced auditory hallucinations, a common symptom of schizophrenia, was at the American Psychiatric Association meeting in San Diego in 1997. A pharmaceutical company was demonstrating an audiotape they had developed. Seated in a sound-proof booth, wearing headphones, I was subjected to stereo hallucinations which seemed to come from every direction inside my head. At the same time I was trying to take part in a mock interview. The experience was both eerie and fascinating. It was extremely difficult to concentrate on the interviewer's questions, never mind organise a coherent answer, while being constantly interrupted by unpredictable voices and noises. For the first time in 15 years of practising psychiatry I had an inkling of what it must be like to be psychotic and hallucinating. It was a great learning experience and should be mandatory for anyone working with people suffering from schizophrenia or other forms of psychosis.

The technology will go much further than this, however. I can see a time in maybe ten to twenty years when it will be possible, using information technology and virtual reality techniques, to almost perfectly recreate many medical and psychiatric disorders in cyberspace. A patient with, say, early symptoms of epilepsy, alzheimers disease, depression or schizophrenia will join their doctor in a virtual reality "booth". The doctor will be able to recreate the patient's exact symptoms using virtual reality techniques to help in diagnosing and monitoring the disorder. Doctors won't have to rely on verbal descriptions of symptoms and their own observations of patients' behaviour as they do at present. These booths are already being built. I recently spent some time in the million dollar "cave", as it is called, at the University of Michigan in Ann Arbor. The diagnostic possibilities of combining virtual reality approaches to diagnosis with the connectivity and power of Internet 2 are almost limitless.

Affective computing — computers have feelings, too

Far-fetched as it sounds, it is already possible for information to be electrically passed along a line of people holding hands with terminals attached to the legs of the person at each end of the line. This sounds weird, but we all know that we transmit electricity and must wear rubber shoes when repairing electrical equipment. It is therefore logical, even if it seems unreal right now, that we could literally be a part of the information system. Dr Andy Lippman from the Massachusetts Institute of Technology Media Laboratory, who describes himself as a "digital futurist", has described this future of "affective computing" — computing with feelings.

What could this mean for patients? If you are depressed, you may have, in a few years time, a "depression monitor" strapped to your arm. On particularly bad days the monitor could transmit a message to your doctor letting him or her know to contact you. Perhaps this will be the sort of technology that will help prevent suicides.

Such technology is not in the realms of fantasy. Already people are wearing cardiac monitors which are linked to 24-hour central monitoring services. If the gauges look abnormal the service rings the patient, or in some instances, sends an ambulance out. Suicidal depression is as much an emergency as heart failure, and hopefully in the future it can be monitored. If it can be then lives will be saved.

Every face tells a story — distributed intelligence

Our faces show our emotions. They are the window of our feelings. Clinicians are trained to both consciously and unconsciously pick up diagnostic cues from patients' faces. We know what someone physically looks like when they are depressed, but we can't physiologically describe it. We know that their brow is furrowed, their mouth drawn, their skin looks dry and pasty, they are tearful and their face moves slowly. Soon we will be able to mathematically measure and model our facial features by converting a video to digital data. Visual diagnostic tests will also be used to assess strokes, neurological movement disorders, even side-effects of medication. And much more accurately than we can do so at present.

These visual X-rays will be combined with simple facial sensors, such as are already being used by Dr Dave Warner (1997), another futurist, who works at the Institute for Interventional Informatics in San Diego. He believes that we will eventually have multi-media patient records that particularly concentrate on patients' faces. These will give us objective information to assist in patient care. And of course patients will be able to use sensors at home to give them more control over their treatment options. Meanwhile Dr Rick Satava (1996),

Professor of Surgery at Yale, talks of a three-dimensional model of the human body, with multiple MRI scans showing internal physical details and digitised pictures showing the outside. This is the ultimate visual medical record. Although it is still some years away, I am sure it will happen.

Are we close to utopia?

Before we get too self congratulatory, let us pause for a moment. There is no point in being clever enough to invent all these new technologies if we don't use them properly.

Ervin Duggan, the chief executive officer of the Public Broadcasting Service in the United States, believes that many of us are guilty of "techno-Utopianism" — excessive, uncritical acceptance of technologies. He believes that worshippers of techno-Utopia don't use the new technologies as effectively as they could because they view the technologies as ends in themselves rather than tools. He suggests that every technology "implies habits of the mind", and, using television as an example, says that it has led us to concentrate on superficial, rapid acquisition of knowledge rather than deep thinking, careful consideration.

It is also important that we do not allow fabulous technologies to be overshadowed by the sort of commercialism evident on cable TV channels, where 30-second news bites and trivia have replaced serious consideration of important issues. It is essential that patients and clinicians drive the development of e-health, not advertisers, the media, business or "technologies in search of an application".

On a more positive note, Warner (1997) has this to say:

As an information bank the Internet has massively fostered an awareness of human health and the possibilities for its improvement. Medicine on the global information highway is not just going to be reserved for the type of practitioner who comes from a Western medical school and was trained in a hospital. The content will be profoundly diverse. There is no precedent for medicine in cyberspace. Everything from basic vitamin approaches to acupuncture, homoeopathy, psychic healing, past life regression and psychedelic shamanism are flourishing to one degree or another.

And he is optimistic about the future of health online:

Out of these ideas and with this technology there will emerge a culture of medical Cybernauts committed to creating a world of healthy individuals, families and communities, enhancing the quality of life.

E-healthcare promises huge benefits for patients, clinicians and society in general. But in embracing the technology, the human factor must not be forgotten. It is not the cleverness of the technology that is important but how we use it to derive the most benefit for everyone. We have to learn to improve, to control, and to effectively use the tools and techniques discussed in this book in order to improve our health and to enrich the quality of our lives.

In this world there are those who make things happen, those who watch what happens and those who wonder what happened. Let us all make e-healthcare happen, and happen well.

INFORMATION AND SITES ON THE INTERNET

This is a quick guide to useful websites and to general information about the Internet. Remember to use the search strategies described in Chapter 4 if you are looking for specific information. They will increase your chance of efficiently finding reliable information sources.

1. Learning the Internet

A few points:

- The Internet has approximately 300 million users worldwide (as of May 2000), with over 3.5 trillion email messages sent annually.
- By the year 2002 there will be 500 million Internet users.
- The number of websites is doubling every 53 days.
- Currently there are over 100,000 health-related websites.
- A new network joins the Internet every 30 minutes.
- Forty per cent of the general population in the United States over age 16 make use of the Internet — about 70 million adults.
- Of the 70 million about one-third retrieve health and medical information.
- Between 60 and 80 per cent of physicians in the United States, the United Kingdom and Australia are connected to the Internet.

A simple interactive course which teaches you how to use the Internet can be found at http://www.netskills.ac.uk/TONIC/. It includes some simple work-based tutorials and is a good place to start from.

2. Searching the Internet

Professional health Internet searches

There are two major reference libraries worth chasing up for academic publications within the area of health. These are Medline and PsychoInfo.

Medline

http://www.ncbi.nlm.nih.gov

Medline is without doubt the premier medical information search facility in the world, and it is now free on the Internet thanks to a truly generous gesture from the Clinton administration. I have been using this search facility for many years, mainly through libraries, and it is now fantastic to find it so easily accessible. The only problem with Medline is that, because it is so huge, with over 9,000,000 papers being cited and new papers going on all the time from almost 4,000 health-related journals, it tends to be three or four months out-of-date. For most people, however, that is not a real problem. While we're at it this National Library of Medicine website is probably the best single site to access quality health information in the world. Bookmark it.

PsycInfo

http://www.HealthGate.com/res/index.shtml

PsycInfo is the premier psychological-related database and is produced by the American Psychological Association. It covers more than 1300 journals in over 25 languages and has been operating since 1967.

Personalised search engines

One of the beauties of the Internet is that you can define your own searches and have references sent to you on a regular basis on the topic of your choice. You can effectively keep up-to-date with your own personalised electronic newspaper.

NewsPage

http://www.newspage.com/

This is a fairly news-oriented "Internet newspaper". Most of their service is still free, but it looks as if it is going to go commercial in the near future and already some charges are being made. At present over 20 per cent of all of the items tracked on NewsPage relate to health, so it is a good place to visit.

NewsTracker

http://nt.excite.com/

This is the largest of the electronic personalised newspapers. It collects information from over 300 web-based newspapers and magazines each day, and researches them several times a day. NewsTracker includes major newspapers such as the *New York Times*, the *Washington Post* and the *Guardian*, and is very helpful if you are looking for health information that has been published in broadsheets rather than in academic journals.

Google search engine

www.google.com

This is the search engine of choice presently recommended by many librarians. It is a fascinating engine with good linked search strategies. It also has the ability to prioritise websites that receive the heaviest traffic, hence you receive the most popular sites first. And it is huge, with apparently over one billion webpages covered in its searches. You will be amazed at how accurately this engine can find quite obscure information, especially if you don't have all the precise details.

Breaking health news (Reuters)

http://www.reutershealth.com

The international news organisation Reuters has a continuously updated list of current health stories, mainly taken from major medical journals, with sections focused for the consumer (health eLine and for the professional, Medical News). If you want an immediate update on the world's latest health news from the medical journals, this is probably the place to come.

Medical quotations
http://www.acponline.org\medquotes\index.html
If you want to see what famous, or infamous, people have said about your illness, this is a fascinating site, with over 30,000 medical quotations on every conceivable subject. For fun, I looked up "malingering" and was delighted to find a quote from Dr Richard Asher, taken from his book *Talking Sense* (1972): "the pride of a doctor who is called a malingerer is akin to that of a fisherman who has landed an enormous fish, and whose stories (like those of the fisherman) may become somewhat exaggerated in the telling". Asher then followed up with three golden rules for malingering, aimed at such patients: "(1) You must make the impression that you hate to be ill; (2) make up your mind for one disease and stick to it; (3) don't tell the doctor too much".

3. Patient information

This is where we go into information overload — the volume of information available is massive. I have not attempted to quote anything like all the sources. Most of the major Internet service providers, such as Yahoo and America Online, have large health resources that are kept up-to-date and generally comprehensive, so don't hesitate to try them as well as the sites suggested here.

General information

Commercial consumer sites

There are a large number of these, and rather than reviewing them all individually, my advice would be for you to go to http://www.gomez.com and access them from there. The best known of these are sites such as Healtheon/webMD, Doctor Koop.com, Intellihealth, Onhealth, Planet Rx.com, Health Central.com, and America'sDoctor.com. All of these sites offer comprehensive content and have a commercial perspective. Many of them have partnerships with very reputable academic institutions, and on the whole the content is of a reasonable quality. These sites are heavily used on the Internet, mainly because of the large marketing budgets that are devoted to them. They are generally consumer-focused, but the information that they provide has to, of course, be treated with a degree of scepticism, because it is there to support a commercial venture and to ensure that you, or health professionals, regularly visit the site to buy its products or services. Remember that not all sites are run for the right motives. Two organisations in the United States that are combating fraudulent health sites, among others, are the Federal Trade Commission (http://www.ftc.gov) and the Food and Drug Administration (http://www.fda.gov).

Global health network

http://www.pitt.edu/HOME/GHNet/GHNet.html

The global health network from the University of Pittsburgh aims to encourage healthcare professionals and consumers to participate in an international network of information on health, which is dedicated to the prevention of disease in the 21st century as well as to a concurrent reduction in expenditure on health globally. This is a massive and well-organised site with excellent coverage of women's general health and mental health, as well as disaster-related activities.

Prevline (Centre for Substance Abuse Prevention, US Department of Health and Human Services)

http://www.health.org

The mission of the National Clearing House for Alcohol and Drug Information is to provide the world's largest resource for current information concerning substance abuse. They seem to have been successful so far, as this is a massive site with access to over 8,000 prevention-related materials, and searches of various alcohol and drug database bibliographies. There is also access to free or low-cost distribution of over 1,000 items of substance-abuse materials including fact sheets, brochures, pamphlets, posters and videotapes. There is an extraordinary amount of material on this site, including statistics on almost every conceivable aspect of alcohol and drug abuse and information on upcoming conferences and research meetings.

Yahoo health

www.yahoo.com/health

Yahoo's aim is simple: to categorise the complete resources on the Internet of all areas of health. Unfortunately there is no attempt to determine information accuracy or reliability. Hence, while there are a large series of health indexes, many of the sites quoted are dubious in the extreme. Be wary.

"Leaflets" on disorders

http://www.hebs.scot.nhs.uk/

Thousands of leaflets giving simple information for patients on particular disorders or conditions have been produced around the world. Many of these have been collected by a fascinating site from Scotland run by the Scottish Health Education Board.

On the whole the electronic leaflets chosen and edited are simple, straightforward, well written and accurate. Make this a *must* on your Internet visits.

Quackwatch

http://www.quackwatch.com/

This site provides information on all sorts of dubious health practices — fascinating, and sometimes terrifying. If you find any really strange health advice on the net please tell the authors of this site so they can check it out.

Internet mental health

http://www.mentalhealth.com/

Dr Phillip Long, a Canadian psychiatrist, does a great job of keeping this site up-to-date, comprehensive and interesting. There are a number of really important stories from consumers published here, as well as excellent information on all the psychiatric disorders, a series of online diagnostic tests you can do yourself, and a very detailed listing of medications.

The Metanoia website

http://www.metanoia.com

This contains a fascinating combination of practical and philosophical writings on the nature of Internet therapy. It is also designed to allow Internet therapists of all persuasions to show their wares. Have a look at it, but bear in mind the advice on how to select a therapist.

Mining Co Guide to Health Resources

http://www.miningco.com

This site is set up to mine the resources of the Internet for new information. Their regular newsletters are interesting and helpful, and they have a knack of disseminating useful information about new research findings.

Molecular Biology (at the National Centre for Biotechnology Information)
http://www.ncbi.nlm.nih.gov
This authoritative site explains and explores the technical and ethical issues surrounding the exciting field of genomics and the amazing advances occurring in biotechnology. It also allows you to look at the complete genome sequence of the fruit fly (*Drosophila melanogaster*). The full sequence was first described in March 2000 and will give you an idea of what to expect for humans. And while you're there, take the time to look at the amazing databases relevant to the human genome project itself.

Sites for selected health organisations and disorders

Self-help organisations
The easiest way of finding these is through the Charities Aid Foundation at http://www.charitynet.org/main.html. This site details almost 100,000 charities, and many of these are directly related to self-help organisations, and the search facility can find these for you.

Onhealth's homepage
http://www.Onhealth.com
This homepage declares: "We know how critical it is for you to arm yourself with the information you need to make better health decisions and be aggressive advocates for your own health with a bureaucracy that makes you fight for your rights." This seems to be a good source for health information that is regularly updated with healthcare news. It has an interesting section called "A–Z" which provides information about a wide

variety of disorders linking the user to appropriate resources and work support groups directly.

Alzheimers Association

http://www.alz.org

This site was developed by the Alzheimers Association, Chicago. It is a very professional site that aims to provide information to patients, families and carers of people with Alzheimers disease. It also provides support networks for those who are affected by this devastating illness. Alzheimers affects 10 per cent of people over the age of 65 and 20 per cent over the age of 80, and families and caregivers carry enormous burdens, so the site is clearly essential. The information provided is of high quality and the whole site is very impressive.

Sports Medicine

http://www.intelli.com\\vhosts\\aossm-isite\\html

This is an interesting site from the American Orthopedic Society for Sports Medicine. It has a lot of education materials, and, in particular, information about their recent campaign on "boomeritis", a term they have coined to relate to the sports injuries in babyboomers who are overdoing their exercise. So if you want some babyboomer sports injury prevention tips, go to this site.

Nutrition (Centre for Disease Control and Prevention)

http://www.cdc.gov

This site takes a sensible and pragmatic approach to the confusing area of nutrition. We are all human and will all "sin" nutritionally at least occasionally, but here you can be confident of getting high-quality advice about your eating habits.

Health for kids

http://www.kidspsych.org

This is a beautifully animated multimedia site targeted at children to help them explore their health and develop effective problem-solving strategies. The site operates through a series of games featuring Oochina who is equally attractive to adults.

The dermatology online atlas

http://www.dermis.net

Most doctors know very little about dermatology, and skin diseases are often badly treated in practice. At this site you can work your way through an unbelievable number of pictures of skin disorders. Not all the pictures are for the faint-hearted, but they are very useful.

Travellers health information

http://www.cdc.gov\\travel\\

The National Centre for Infectious Diseases has produced a great page on travellers' health. You can select your own part of the world and quickly and easily find out what preventative measures you need to take to remain fit and well while travelling in that region. There is great practical advice on everything from sanitation and immunisation to the best way of reliably treating water to make it safe to drink.

Eyes

http://www.eyenet.org

The American Academy of Ophthalmology has created an interesting site with a large number of resources specifically for patients. Information on everything from cancer of the eye to lens implantation and refractive surgery is discussed. The site is well laid out and appears to be relatively non-commercial.

Cancer
http://www.canceronline.org
This is one of the best health sites on the Internet. It is a great resource for anyone with cancer, and particularly for carers of people with cancer, and provides much more than good-quality information. The difference with Cancer Online is the practical, supportive approach taken to the loved ones of those with cancer, and the collaborative manner in which the clinicians involved in providing cancer care can share their expertise to reach a large number of patients and carers. This is a sensitive, regularly updated site that takes the broadest possible approach to cancer care and which emphasises a sensible holistic approach combining the best of medical and technical care with the appropriate attention to the mind/body continuum. It even has a humour section edited by Sidney Love, a Canadian engineering physicist and also a survivor of prostate cancer. This site, founded by Arlene Harder and Craig Miles, cannot be too highly praised and is a model of excellence on the Internet.

The Ferguson Report
http://www.fergusonreport.com
Dr Tom Ferguson, Associate Professor of Health and Thematics of the University of Texas Health Science Center, was recently recognised by Intel's Internet Health Initiative as one of four pioneering "online health heroes". His reports, published at "unpredictable intervals for active players in the Online Health Revolution", are fascinating. Ferguson, otherwise known as "Doc Tom", is an innovative thinker who takes a strong patient-oriented perspective and predicts that online health resources will produce a major shift in health care. His report is a great place to gain up-to-the-minute information on health happenings on the Internet.

About.com

http://www.about.com

This is one of the most interesting sites on the web, mainly because of the use of "guides" who are from many different backgrounds and over twenty countries. Some are health experts, such as Dr Leonard Holmes, in the mental health field, while many more are consumers or carers. The guide's role is to provide assistance and guidance to users of About.com, to moderate chats and initiate discussions, and to keep their areas of the site as up-to-date as possible. Although there are no absolute guarantees about the quality of content on About.com, it is possible to get replies and genuine assistance from the guides. If you are really keen, you can even become a guide yourself. Health is, of course, only one relatively small section of what is a massive Internet portal covering an extraordinary range of topics.

Family Planning and Population Health (John Hopkins University Center)

http://www.jhuccp.org

This site is a fascinating mix of high-quality information from multiple databases, mainly focused on family planning, HIV/Aids, population, and other related health issues. Apart from the conventional, excellent databases and search engines you might expect from a major university, this site has a very personal feel with daily feature articles (e.g. did you know that over 100 million women around the world now take the pill?) and a fascinating collection of over 3,500 photographs of reproductive health activities around the world which are available for everyone to share and use for health promotion purposes. The Internet links on this site are massive, with over 1100 links available in a searchable format. The immunisation resources hosted here, in conjunction with the Bill and Melinda

Gates children's vaccine program, are extremely comprehensive. This is a great example of an academic site with a human face.

Anaesthesia

Gasnet at http://www.gasnet.org

This is a site primarily developed for health professionals working in anaesthesia, but it has some high-quality information for anyone with an interest in the topic. The site has all the usual access to education materials, journals, discussion lists and information about meetings and societies, but the really valuable part is the virtual anaesthesia textbook which can be accessed through the Internet links section of Gasnet. This is a massive and fascinating virtual textbook that was commenced in 1996 and consists of a large number of Internet links organised by subject into chapters and structured to mimic a general anaesthesia textbook. This global program, coordinated by Dr Chris Thompson from the Royal Prince Alfred Hospital in Sydney, Australia, will teach you everything on anaesthesia from the fundamentals of laser surgery and anaesthesia through to intubation, pain management and how to manage serious poisoning. If you are going under the knife, or simply want information on anything from professional, ethical and historical anaesthetic issues to high-powered pharmacology, then this is a great site.

Alcoholics Anonymous

http://alcoholics-anonymous.org/

This huge site has a lot of interesting information, based on the 12 steps approach to the treatment of alcoholism, and is very focused on consumers.

Schizophrenia
http://www.Schizophrenia.com
This site is without doubt the best site in the world on schizophrenia and is maintained by the self-help organisation of the same name. If you want to learn about this disorder, which affects 1 per cent of the population of the world, then spend some time here. Apart from the carefully presented and well-organised information and links, there are great stories from consumers and an excellent and up-to-date research section.

Suicide
The Suicide Awareness Voice of Education http://www.save.org
This is a comprehensive site giving information on depression and suicide. There are a large number of useful resources available here, many of which can be emailed directly to site visitors. This is a hugely popular service and includes pieces on what to do if someone you know becomes suicidal, frequently asked questions on suicide and depression, and advice for survivors after a loved one has suicided.

Griefnet
http://rivendell.org/
Developed by a Michigan-based, non-profit foundation, this site aims to assist people recovering from grief by providing both information and support groups. The site provides a wide variety of information not only of the conventional variety but also including some heart-rending poems and some helpful thoughts and ideas. One fascinating and unusual feature is the memorial section, where you can actually post a memorial to a loved one. Some of the letters at this site, particularly to lost children, are quite remarkable. Don't look at them without a handkerchief.

Information on medication

It is hard to go past the United States Pharmacopoeia as a source of accurate, detailed and authoritative information on medications. You can find this, and access it easily, through http://www.intelihealth.com/. Simply put in the name of any medication you fancy, either the drug company name or the chemical name, and you will get excellent and immediate information.

Medications are also well covered in many of the sites already listed.

Discussion groups

Anyone can join a list. You simply have to subscribe to the topic of your choice. The only problem with lists is that they can end up flooding your email with multiple messages, because any time anyone sends a message to the list it gets redirected to the emails of everyone else on the list. If you happen to be on a list with many hundreds of other people, this can be a pretty awful experience.

No-one knows exactly how many discussion lists are available through the Internet. I have only personally been a part of three or four, and have usually unsubscribed after a while because of the extraordinary number of messages that started filling up my email intray. If you want to look for the types of lists on the Internet, and there are probably now well over 100,000, go to the directory of mailing lists data base at http://www.liszt.com. Discussion lists will gradually change over the next few years, and already it is becoming possible to simply get sent lists of discussion topics, rather than every individual email to the list, so that email overload doesn't occur so quickly.

4. Online health resources

There are many good health information sites on the Internet. The site for the Centre for Online Health at the University of Queensland (http://www.coh.uq.edu.au) has been developed as a very broad health and information technology site where you can access the majority of health/IT journals in the world and which contains a meta search engine allowing you to easily find almost all relevant references with reasonable ease. Another notable site is the Telemedicine Information Exchange at http://tie.telemed.org in Portland, Oregan. This site is run by the Telemedicine Research Centre which is funded by the US federal government to provide a constant library of sources on telemedicine. The site has a great reference list and is very helpful.

There are three main telemedicine journals, all of which have an online presence.

1. The Journal of Telemedicine and Telecare (http://www.coh.uq.edu.au) is edited by Professor Richard Wootton of the University of Queensland, Australia, and published by the Royal Society of Medicine in London. It was the first academic telemedicine journal to be referenced by Medline and has a truly global view.
2. The Telemedicine Journal (http:www.liebertpub.com/tmj) is published by the American Telemedicine Association (http://www.atmeda.org) and edited by Professor Rashid Bashshur from the University of Michigan. It is primarily focused on American telemedicine and contains a wide variety of excellent papers.
3. Telemedicine Today (http://www.telemedtoday.com) has been instrumental in facilitating the rapid development of telemedicine around the world as a quality forum allowing interaction between clinicians, vendors, patients and information technology experts.

The majority of health informatics journals can be accessed through http://www.coh.uq.edu.au.

5. Professional sites/organisations

The following professional sites are also useful for patients.

Medscape homesite

http://www.medscape.com

Medscape describes itself as "an interactive, multi-specialty, commercial Web service for clinicians and consumers". This service is free, although a user has to take out a one-time membership registration. The site has a large number of useful facilities, including an extensive searchable database of peer-reviewed clinical articles and unrestricted free access to Medline and the national drug database. The site includes a large number of daily medical news items as well as an online bookstore and free subscription to *Med pulse*, Medscape's weekly email newsletter.

Health on the Internet

http://www.hon.ch/

This site is run by a non-profit organisation whose vision is "realising the benefits of the Internet and related technologies in the fields of medicine and health care". The organisation has developed a Health on the Net logo for its pages and is attempting to use it as a quality-control marker for health science in general. Although there are no formal standards on the Internet, the Health on the Net principles are being increasingly quoted and recognised.

Medical Matrix

http://www.medmatrix.org/index.asp

This huge site has links to over 4,000 Internet sites which are said to have been assessed for their quality, with some gaining merit stars as being "best of specialty". Like many sites, this one has a simple online registration form. Don't be put off by this. It is well worth registering and it won't cost you anything.

CliniWeb

http://www.ohsu.edu/cliniweb

This is a pointedly professional site which is attempting to provide information only for "health care education or practice". It does, however, provide accurate and fairly targeted searches and is well worth using.

The Doctor's Internet Handbook

http://www.roysocmed.ac.uk/handbook.htm

This is the webpage that goes with a great little book by Robert Kiley entitled *The Doctor's Internet Handbook*. My view is that this book should be mandatory reading for all doctors and most health-care professionals, as it gives such a good, simple guide to the Internet and many Internet resources. The beauty of the website is that it has hotlinks to all of the sites quoted in the book, and it is certainly one of my key references. Although the book and the site are focused towards doctors, if you want to learn about the Internet quickly and easily, buy this book or check out the links on this site.

The University of Iowa Virtual Hospital

http://australia.vh.org

The Virtual Hospital is a tremendous project, a digital health scientist's library, which is a great health reference and health promotion tool for both patients and clinicians. The site has user-friendly and reliable information for both patients and health-care providers and a huge list of resources about common health problems in adults. You can learn about everything from vomiting and toothache to cancer and HIV at this thoroughly professional site.

Virtual medical textbooks

http://www.emedicine.com

This a fascinating site that professes to involve 6,000 or more physicians from around the world in a massive undertaking to write a series of virtual medical textbooks. The site is heavily sponsored by a large number of commercial and non-commercial organisations, but has clear guidelines about the sponsorship, with the quote "sponsors do not influence content" on every page. Although these textbooks, covering all possible areas of health, are primarily intended for health professionals, they are an extraordinarily comprehensive source of information for consumers. There is one section on "consumer treatment guidelines" which is probably the weakest part of the site, as these are rather static and hard to relate to as an individual; but the information for health professionals is generally superb and is worth downloading to have with you to discuss with your doctor in person. If nothing else, tell your doctor about this site. Watch out for the fascinating three-dimensional computerised atlas of the human body, the visible human project, shown on this site. If you want to literally look at your inner self, this is the best place to come.

Ethics on the Web (through the Internet Healthcare Coalition)

http://www.ihealthcoalition.org

This site declares its mission to be the provision of quality health-care resources on the Internet, and is a non-profit coalition with a high profile board of directors from both industry and public sectors. Its main work to date appears to have been the development of an e-health code of ethics which is very sensible and well worth viewing.

Ethics of Health Care (University of Pennsylvania Center for Bioethics)

http://www.bioethics.net

The Center for Bioethics defines bioethics as the study of the moral implications of science, medicine and research, and this site gives a balanced view of many of the difficult ethical issues facing patients and health-care practitioners around the world. In an area where philosophical or religious views can predominate, bioethics.net examines the moral implications of topics such as assisted suicide, abortion, cloning and organ transplantation. The site is attractively set up with interesting "breaking news" stories and a comprehensive, relevant virtual library and set of links. There has been a particularly interesting recent discussion on the ethical rights of Internet users breaking all the typical rules of "netiquette" in what is in reality an "unrestrained medium for communication" — the Web.

HealthWeb

http://www.healthweb.org

This is a well-organised not-for-profit site set up by a variety of medical centres in the mid-west of the United States. It has a large number of carefully researched resources described under a long list of subjects. The downside to this site is that most of the resources quoted are American, but they are generally reputable.

Multimedia health resources (Martindale's Health Science Guide)

www-sci.lib.uci.edu/HSG/HSGuide.html

Do you want to know how to calculate your biorhythms? Or your life expectancy? Perhaps you would rather know your risk of getting breast cancer or the average cost of dental care in your home town. On this site, which was started in 1994 and is hosted in the University of California, Irvine, there are over 60,000 teaching files, 125,000 medical cases, 1100 courses/textbooks, 1500 tutorials, 3700 databases and 10,000 movies. I haven't attempted to look at all of them, but found the over 11,000 "medical calculators" a fascinating, if mind-boggling, resource.

Selected professional health associations and journals

The World Health Organisation at http://www.who.int is the best site if you want to get a good overview of global healthcare. The information provided is of high quality, and generally relates to global health policies. The recently released "World Health Report 2000" is downloadable, and through this report you can take a helicopter view of health around the world. It focuses on the problems in our present health systems, and the need for reforms and improvements. It can be heavy going but the statistics are fascinating. Also look at the American Medical Association: www.ama-assn.org

Almost all major medical journals are now represented on the Internet. The following are examples:

New England Journal of Medicine: http://www.nejm.org/

Journals of the American Medical Association: http://jama.ama-assn.org

British Medical Journal: http://www.bmj.com

The Lancet: http://www.thelancet.com/

Other quality evaluated subject gateways

Healthfinder
http://www.healthfinder.gov
This is the official United States consumer health gateway which provides access to almost 6,000 reliable resources from the federal government and public and private sector partners. The support groups linked to this site are generally affiliated with credible organisations, and the site also links to carefully selected resources that are offered by commercial sites. Healthfinder is one of the biggest health information sites in the world, attracting about a million visitors per month, and its 20 hot topics and the daily health news are great for those who wish to keep completely up-to-date. Healthfinder is well laid out, is easy to navigate, and has a very suave look and feel.

NHS Direct (National Health Service Direct — United Kingdom)
http://www.nhsdirect.nhs.uk
This is the British equivalent of Healthfinder — a high-quality, carefully managed site providing health information for consumers. The most interesting aspects of this site are the number of simple guides provided to allow you to explore common symptoms. The guides are in the form of decision trees which you can work through, and they cover many topics, from headaches to itchy rashes. The site strongly encourages self-care, by giving you the resources to make appropriate decisions, and also allowing you immediate telephone access to a 24-hour, 7 days a week nursing telephone service. Perhaps the most sensible advice I could find on the site related to ways in which you could work out whether your baby was ill, an important problem that confronts all parents.

OMNI

http://omni.ac.uk

This site is the United Kingdom's gateway to high-quality biomedical Internet resources. All resources meet the quality criterion as defined by the OMNI Advisory Group for Evaluation Criteria. Another important site for you to bookmark.

Medical Matrix

http://www.medmatrix.org/

Aimed primarily at United States physicians and health workers, Medical Matrix ranks Internet resources based on their utility for point-of-care clinical application. Quality, peer review, full content, multimedia features and unrestricted access are emphasised in the rankings.

Gomez.com — the e-commerce authority

http://www.gomez.com

Gomez.com may well become one of the most influential health sites on the Internet. The mission of Gomez is to be the "premier provider of e-commerce decision support and online customer experience measurement". Gomez has recently moved into health, and as well as providing consumer ratings of books, furniture, banks and the like now also provides ratings of health content, or portal, sites, online pharmacies (for prescriptions) and e-commerce sites with a health emphasis, as well as the top "Internet cholesterol information" sites. It is particularly interesting to see how the many, mainly commercial, health-content sites rank when compared with each other. If you want to quickly find a question and answer doctor on the Internet, this site is probably the best place to come for a comprehensive selection.

6. Other databases

Cochrane Reviews

http://www.update-software.com/cochrane-frame.html

This is the best single source of reliable evidence about the effects of health care and the use of "evidence based medicine". Abstracts are available without charge and the information given is guaranteed to be of the highest quality because of the exhaustive process of peer review and scientific analysis that all Cochrane Review papers undergo. Subscription is required to read the full text of the reviews, but most good health libraries will have these available on CD-Rom. This site is intended for professionals and most of the reviews are highly technical, especially from a statistical perspective, but print out the ones you are interested in and discuss them with your doctor in person. No doctor should ever object to you bringing in a Cochrane Review — these are the ultimate in evidence-based medical reports.

7. Guidelines and questions

These are your best set of signposts to follow to determine whether you are getting therapy in accord with the best clinical and research findings. Try http://www.guidelines.gov/index.asp for a comprehensive list of guidelines. Similarly, if you want massive lists of frequently asked questions, go to http://www.faqs.org.

8. The future of health on the Internet

No-one is sure what the future of health on the Internet holds, but these sites will give you some ideas:

Next generation Internet initiative: http://www.ngi.gov/apps/

The Internet 2 program: www.Internet2.edu
The G8 healthcare initiative: http://www.ehto.be/sp5

GLOSSARY

Analogue: Any form of information, usually electronic, that is created and transmitted as a continuous stream. It includes wave forms from oscilloscopes, standard photographs and most x-rays. Modems are used to convert digital computer data to an analogue form in order to be able to transmit it over ordinary telephone lines.

Asynchronous communication: Communication that takes place in different timeframes according to the user's convenience (e.g. email).

Bandwidth: The capacity of an electronic "pipe" to transmit data per unit of time. Typically the higher the bandwidth the more data or information that can be transmitted. Usually measured in kilobits per second (kbps) or megabits per second (mbps).

Bit: The basic unit of information used by computers for information entry, transmission and storage. The information is stored in **b**inary dig**it** form as a series of zeros and ones.

Broadband: Generally refers to high bandwidth sufficient to support real-time videoconferencing or fast data downloads.

Browser: A software program that allows you to access the World Wide Web. Most people use Netscape or Internet Explorer.

Byte: Simply a data character, such as a single letter or number, that is made up of eight bits. Megabytes are units of storage essentially defining the numbers of characters that can be stored on a disk or computer.

Call centre: Computer-enabled telephone centres that are becoming increasingly important in health. They are often staffed by health professionals and may be used to provide information for patients, as well as for telephone assessments of our health.

Codec: The electronic device that converts and compresses electronic signals to allow them to be transmitted through relatively small communication pipes. The term comes from **Co**der/**dec**oder.

Compressed video: Video images that have been simplified to remove redundant information, thereby reducing the amount of bandwidth required to transmit them.

Consultation: The event that occurs when a doctor, or other clinician, provides their expert services to a patient for a specific purpose.

Cyberspace: An increasingly popular term to describe the notional information "space" that is created between computer networks.

Diagnosis: The process of categorising a patient, or their symptoms and signs, as well as laboratory results, to decide the nature of a disease process.

Digital: Information coded in discrete numerical values, bits. A digital data stream is simply made up of zeros and ones (the bits) and can be integrated and manipulated more easily with other data streams because it is so simple.

Download: To retrieve a file from another computer and copy it on to your own.

Effectiveness: In the health-care arena, the degree to which an intervention, or treatment, produces a measurable increase in a person's health-care state.

Electronic medical record: Also known as the CPR (computerised patient record), EHR (electronic health record) or EPR (electronic patient record), it is a term that is generally used to describe computer-based patient record systems. These systems often also include the ability to enter orders for medications and tests, and may be linked to billing programs.

Email: Electronic mail which is the messaging system that is available to your computer network.

Encryption: The mathematical scrambling of a file or data stream so that it cannot be deciphered at the receiving end without a correct key to the scrambled code. This is a simple privacy feature.

FAQ: Frequently asked questions that appear on websites, usually with common responses.

Firewall: A security barrier that is erected between the Internet and any local private computer network, an intranet. It prevents communication between the two and is particularly important in the health-care arena to prevent confidential health-information about individuals becoming widely available to the rest of the world.

Flame: An angry, often abusive, message sent on the Internet.

Hard drive: The internal storage device on your computer which saves files, data and programs.

Health: This has been defined by the World Health Organization as a "complete state of physical, mental and social wellbeing". Unfortunately, very few of us reach this ideal.

Health care: The activities that are intended to maintain our health, either on an individual or a community basis.

Hit: A single access of a website.

Home page: Your own Internet site written in HTML.

Hypertext: The highlighted section of text that you see on a webpage which allows you to retrieve a linked document.

Hypertext markup language: This is commonly known as HTML and is a simple system of codes that are used to construct Web homepages.

Internet: A loose aggregration of many thousands of individual computers and computer networks, which form an enormous world-wide area network.

Intranet: Effectively a "private Internet" which uses the same communications protocols as the Internet, but is only accessible to an agreed set of computers.

IP address: The address of a computer on the Internet which is managed through its Internet Provider and allows the computer to receive and send messages.

ISDN: The Integrated Services Digital Network, which uses digital lines to transmit data instead of the usual analogue lines that are available for most phone calls. This is what is typically used for videoconferencing.

ISP: The **I**nternet **S**ervice **P**rovider is the company or organisation that acts as your gateway to the Internet.

Modem: This term comes from **mo**dulator/**dem**odulator, which is simply an electronic device that transforms digital data from computers to analogue wave forms so that this data can be transmitted over standard phone lines. Most modems now work at a rate of 28 kps, although 56 kps is becoming more common.

Multimedia email: Electronic mail that allows the transmission of not only text but also audio, still images and video.

Network: An assortment of electronic devices, such as computers, printers and scanners, which may be connected using either wires or wireless systems to other devices to allow information exchange.

Offline: Refers to time spent preparing documents or files which can then be sent electronically after connecting to a network.

Online: Refers to time that you spend connected to any form of active computer network linking up with other computers.

Outcome: In the health field, this means the results or measurements of change in health after a particular treatment or intervention.

Pots: The conventional analogue telephone service — Plain Old Telephone Service.

Prevention: Any action in the health field that is taken to prevent a particular activity from occurring. Examples include the use of darkened computer screens to prevent headaches in users or major advertising campaigns to prevent young people from taking up smoking.

Search engine: A site or service on a site that indexes itself and makes the results available to other sites for searching.

Server: A specific computer on a network that is used to store commonly required resources or files. Any Internet sites, or homepages, are stored on the servers of Internet Service Providers.

Store and forward: A mode of transmission for data that has been already saved on a computer hard drive, such as images of patients using a digital camera, which may then be transmitted electronically to wherever required.

Synchronous communication: Communication that takes place in real time (e.g. telemedicine). This is also known as "real time" communication.

TCP/IP: The most popular standard protocols used in data networks around the world today. TCP/IP stands for **T**ransmission **C**ontrol **P**rotocol/**I**nternet **P**rotocol. The TCP is the underlying protocol that servers use to communicate, while the IP is what is used to direct, or route, packets of data on a network.

Telecommunications: The use of wire, radio, fibre or other channels to transmit or receive signals for data, voice or video communication.

Telehealth: A broader term than telemedicine, and generally used for any health delivery system providing health-related activities at a distance.

Telemedicine: The World Health Organization defines this as "the delivery of health care services by health care professionals using information technologies for the exchange of valid information for diagnosis and prevention of disease and injuries, and for the continuing education of health providers as well as research and evaluation, all in the interest of improving the health of individuals and their communities". Telemedicine usually refers to videoconferencing, and this is how the term is used in this book.

Telemetry: The monitoring and study at a distance of our physiological functions, typically heart rate or blood pressure.

Therapeutic intervention: An intervention by a clinician for the purpose of treatment, generally intended to improve a patient's health.

Transmission rate: The amount of information per unit of time that a technology can transmit.

URL: The Uniform Resource Locator, which is the addressing system used on the Internet, to identify a website. The URL tells the Web browser which computer to connect to, and where on that computer the required webpage can be found.

Videoconferencing: The connection of different locations via video camera and monitors which allows everyone to speak to each other and see each other simultaneously. It is often combined, on a desktop, with the ability to pass data across to and from all participants.

Video phone: A small video appliance which attaches to the standard phone system allowing both audio and video communications.

Virtual reality: A simulated environment created on, and with, computers, within which humans are able to interact in an approximation to the real world.

World Wide Web: The Web (WWW) essentially acts as a global publishing system and is a powerful Internet tool for retrieving and distributing information. It uses hypertext links to create a global system of linking pages of information together.

REFERENCES AND FURTHER READING

The following list of references is a combination of those quoted in this book and others that I believe will be of particular interest to readers who wish to explore some of the issues raised in this book in more depth.

Ainsworth, M. Online therapy. http://www.cmhc.com/guide/cyber/

Allen, A. and Grigsby, B. 1998. Consultation activity in 35 specialties. Telemedicine Today. October. pp. 18–19.

Allen, A., Cristoferi, A., Campana, S. and Grimaldi, A. 1997. An Italian telephone-mediated home monitoring service: TeSAN Personal Emergency Response System & Teleservices. Telemedicine Today. December. pp. 25–33.

Amenta, F., Dauri, A. and Rizzo, N. 1998. Telemedicine and medical care to ships without a doctor on board. Journal of Telemedicine and Telecare. Vol. 4. Supp. 1. pp. 44–45.

Asher, R. 1972. Talking Sense. p. 145. Baltimore University Press. Baltimore.

Baer, L., Cukor, P. and Jenike, M. et al. 1995. Pilot studies of telemedicine for patients with obsessive-compulsive disorder. American Journal of Psychiatry. September. 152(9).

Balas, E. Andrew, Jaffrey, F. and Kuperman, G. J. et al. 1997. Electronic communication with patients — evaluation of distance medicine technology. Journal of the American Medical Association, 9 July. Vol. 278. No. 2.

Balch, D. C., Warner, D. J. and Gustke, S. S. 1999. Medical knowledge on demand. Highlights from the third DMI Conference. MD Computing. March–April. 16(20). pp. 48–50.

Ball, C. et al. 1998. Videoconferencing and the hard of hearing. Journal of Telemedicine and Telecare. 4. pp. 57–59.

Ball, C. and Puffett, A. 1998. The assessment of cognitive function in the elderly using videoconferencing. Journal of Telemedicine and Telecare. Vol. 4. Supp. 1. pp. 36–38.

Bashshur, R. 1997. Clinical issues in telemedicine. Telemedicine Journal. Vol. 3. No. 2.

Brosnan, M. 1998. Technophobia: the psychological impact of information technology. Routledge: London.

Cairncross, F. 1997. The death of distance: how the communications revolution will change our lives. Harvard Business School Press: Harvard.

Coeira, E. 1997. Guide to medical informatics, the Internet and telemedicine. Oxford University Press: Oxford.

Colon, Y. Chatter(er)ing through the fingertips: doing group therapy online. http://www.echonyc.com/~women/Issue17/public-colon.html

Doolittle et al. 1998. Hospice care using home-based telemedicine systems. Journal of Telemedicine and Telecare Vol. 4, Supp. 1. pp. 58–59.

Doolittle, G. 1997. A POTS-based tele-hospice project in Missouri. Telemedicine Today. August.

Ferguson, T. 1998. Digital doctoring — opportunities and challenges in electronic patient–physician communication. Journal of the American Medical Association. 21 October. Vol. 280. No. 15. pp. 1361–62.

Gammon, D., Sorlie, T., Bergvik, S. and Sorensen Hoifodt, T. 1998. Psychotherapy supervision conducted by videoconferencing: a qualitative study of users' experiences. Journal of Telemedicine and Telecare. Vol 4. Supp. 1. pp. 33–35.

Gray, J. et al. 1998. Telematics in the neonatal ICU and beyond: improving care, communication and information sharing. Medinfo. 9. pt. 1. pp. 294–97.

Gray, J., Pompilio-Weitzner, G., Jones, P. C., Wang, Q., Coriat, M. and Safran, C. 1998. Baby-care link: development and implementation of a WWW system for neo-natal home telemedicine. Proceedings of the AMIA Symposium. pp. 351–55.

Grohol, J. 1999. The insider's guide to mental health resources online. The Guilford Press: New York.

Gwinnell E. 1998. Online seductions: Falling in love with strangers on the Internet. Kodansha America Inc., New York.

Hodges, L. F. et al. Graphics, Visualisation and Usability Centre, College of Computing, Georgia Tech. www.cc.gatech.edu

Itzhak, B., Weinberger, T., Berkovitch, E. and Reis, S. 1998. Telemedicine in primary care in Israel. Journal of Telemedicine and Telecare. Vol. 4. Supp. 1. pp. 11–14.

Kane, B. and Sands, D. Z. 1998. Guidelines for the clinical use of electronic mail with patients. Journal of the American Medical Informatics Association. Vol. 5. No. 1. January/February.

Kraut, R. Patterson, M., Lundmark, V., Keisler, S., Mukopadhyay, T. and Scherlis, W. 1998. Internet paradox. A social technology that reduces social involvement and psychological well-being? American Psychologist. September. 53(9). pp. 1017–31.

Malaysian Multimedia Supercorridor at www.mdc.com.my

Marks, I. M., Baer, L., Greist, J. H. et al. 1998. CIMH: home self-assessment and self-treatment of obsessive compulsive disorder using a manual and a computer-conducted telephone interview. I: Two UK–US Studies. British Journal of Psychiatry. 172. pp. 406–12. http://www.ex.ac.uk/cimh/btstep.htm

McInnes, A. The agency of the infozone: exploring the effects of a community network. http://www.firstmonday.dk/issues/issues2_2/mcinnes/index.html

Murray, C. J. and Lopez, A. D. (eds) 1996. The global burden of disease: a comprehensive assessment of mortality and disability from diseases, injuries and risk factors in 1990 and projected to 2020. Harvard School of Public Health: Harvard.

National Board for Certified Counselors 1998. NBCC Standards for the Ethical Practice of Webcounseling. http://www.nbcc.org/ethics/wcstandards.htm

Newman, M. G., Consoli, A. and Barr Taylor, C. 1997. Computers in assessment and cognitive behavioral treatment of clinical disorders: anxiety as a case in point. Behavior Therapy. 28. pp. 211–235.

Newman, M. G., Kenardy, J., Herman, S. and Taylor, C. B. 1997.

Comparison of palm-top computer-assisted brief cognitive behavioral treatment to cognitive behavioral treatment of panic disorder. Journal Consultation Clinical Psychology. February 65(1). pp. 178–83.

Oakley-Browne, M. A. and Toole, S. 1996. Computerised self-care programs for depression and anxiety disorders. WHO.

Perednia, D. 1995. Telemedicine technology and clinical applications. Journal of the American Medical Association. 8 February. Vol. 273. No. 6.

Polauf, J. 1998. Psychotherapy on the Internet — theory and technique. http://www.nyreferrals.com/psychotherapy/

Powell, T. 1998. Online counseling: a profile and descriptive analysis. http://netpsych.com/Powell.htm

Rosen, E. 1997. Current uses of desktop telemedicine. Telemedicine Today. March/April.

Rosen, E. 1998. Personal telemedicine. Telemedicine Today. February. pp. 10–13.

Rosen, L. D. and Weil, M. M. 1997. Technostress: coping with mailto:technology@work@home@play. John Wiley and Sons: New York.

Rothchild, E. 1997. E-mail therapy. American Journal of Psychiatry. 154(10). pp. 1476–77.

Satava, R. M. and Jones, S. B. 1996. Virtual reality and telemedicine: exploring advanced concepts. Telemedicine Journal. Fall 2(3). pp. 195–200.

Slack, W. 1997. Cybermedicine. Jossey-Bass: San Francisco.

Smith, R. 1997. The future of healthcare systems. British Medical Journal. 314 (7093). pp. 1495–96.

Spielberg, A. R. 1998. On call and online — sociohistorical, legal, and ethical implications of e-mail for the patient–physician relationship. Journal of the American Medical Association. 21 October. Vol. 280. No. 15.

Stofle, G. Thoughts about online psychotherapy: ethical and practical considerations. http://members.aol.com/stofle/onlinepsych.htm

Suler, J. 1996. The psychology of cyberspace. www1.rider.edu and http://www.behaviour.net

Swartz, D. 1997. Healthcare moves to the Web. Telemedicine Today. December. pp. 36–37.

Van der Weyden, M. 1998. Email: editors, doctors and patients. Medical Journal of Australia. 7–21 December. 169(11–12). pp. 571–72.

Viire, Erik. 1994. A survey of medical issues and virtual reality technology. Virtual Reality World. July/August. pp. 16–20.

Warner, D. J. 1997. The globalization of interventional informatics through Internet mediated distributed medical intelligence. Paper — Pulsar website.

Whitten, P., Collins, B. and Mair, F. 1998. Nurse and patient reactions to a developmental home telecare system. Journal of Telemedicine and Telecare. Vol. 4. No. 3. pp. 152–60.

Wootton, R. et al. 1998. A joint US–UK study of home telenursing. Journal of Telemedicine and Telecare. Vol. 4. Supp. 1. pp. 83–85.

Wootton, R. and Darkins, A. Telemedicine and the doctor–patient relationship. Journal of the Royal College of Physicians. London. November–December 31(6). pp. 598–99.

Wright, D. 1998. Telemedicine and developing countries. Journal of Telemedicine and Telecare. Vol. 4. Supp. 2. pp. 1–88.

Wyatt, J. and Keen, J. 1998. The NHS's new information strategy. http://www.bmj.com/cgi/content/full/317/7163/900

Yale University School of Medicine Department of Surgery. The NASA Commercial Space Center at Yale University Medical Informatics & Technology Applications (MITA). http://Yalesurgery.med.yale.edu/CSC/mita.htm

Yatim, L. 1997. An Israeli telenursing call center: home cardiac telemonitoring: revisiting Israel's Shahal. Telemedicine Today. December. pp. 26–33.

Yellowlees, P. 1997. Successful development of telemedicine systems — seven core principles. Journal of Telemedicine and Telecare. Vol. 3. pp. 215–22.

Yellowlees, P. M. 2000. E-therapy — your guide to mental health in cyberspace. Self-published at www.mightywords.com

Yellowlees, P. M. and Brooks, P. 1999. Health online — the future isn't what it used to be. Medical Journal of Australia. November. Vol. 171. pp. 522–25.

Young, K. 1998. Caught in the net: how to recognize the signs of internet addiction. John Wiley and Sons: New York.

Young, K. The Centre for On-Line Addiction. http://www.netaddiction.com